SILVER SPARKS

Thoughts on Growing Older, Wiser, and Happier

MEG SELIG

First Printing: August, 2020
Nevertheless Press
St. Louis, Mo.

ISBN (paperback): 978-1-64184-419-2
ISBN (e-book): 978-1-64184-420-8
Library of Congress Control Number:

Book and Cover design by JETLAUNCH
Author photo by Rachel Carr

This book is not intended as a substitute for medical advice. For help with specific health issues, contact qualified medical providers. For help with mental health issues, consult a licensed therapist or psychiatrist. You can also get direct help or a referral from the National Suicide Prevention Lifeline: 800-273-8255.

Dedication

This is dedicated to the ones I love:

Thanks, Beth, Trond, and Eloise.
Thanks, Brian.

CONTENTS

PREFACE

"I didn't get old on purpose. It just happened.
If you're lucky, it could happen to you."

—Andy Rooney

I could never have imagined that "older age" could be such a happy time until I started becoming older myself. And I am not alone in my happiness. Surveys reveal that most people over 50 **do** become happier as they age, despite the inevitable health and personal losses that accompany getting older.

Unfortunately, the link between happiness and aging is rarely part of the conversation. As a result, many people dread getting older. The gallows humor in greeting cards for decade birthdays, starting as soon as age 30, testifies to that. We are afraid both of aging itself and of being labeled "old." In fact, there is a newly-coined word for "the fear of aging:" "gerontophobia."

One of my main goals in writing *Silver Sparks: Thoughts on Growing Older, Wiser, and Happier* is to help people of all ages become less afraid of growing older. In the book, I emphasize the fulfilling side of aging, the side that is often ignored in the jokes, inaccurate images, and myths about old age. Not that growing older is all unicorns and butterflies. But the many sources of purpose, pleasure, and pride in the later years often make up for the challenges we face.

Those challenges are real and often seem overwhelming. But with creativity and problem-solving, many "unsolvable" problems can be resolved or bettered in one way or another. To this end, I offer suggestions and ideas for overcoming typical obstacles to happiness in the older years. For example, you'll find chapters on maintaining self-confidence as you age, science-based tips for a healthier body and brain, and how to bounce back from aging crises. I've also ventured into tough subjects like easing the fear of death and finding purpose as you age.

I spent a lot of time thinking about a title. In the end, I chose *Silver Sparks* because it is both optimistic and realistic. "Sparks" remind us of the many flashes of joy, insight, love, and laughter that make our lives meaningful and keep us going during our dark days. "Silver" reminds us of our graying hair, of the storm clouds with their silver linings, and of the precious metal which, even when slightly tarnished, is flexible, useful, and beautiful—just like we are as we age.

To this project I bring my work experiences as a licensed professional counselor, my retirement career as an author and blogger, and my life experiences as a mother, wife, divorcee, grandmother, partner, and friend. *Silver Sparks* includes my blogs on aging from PsychologyToday.com, along with personal essays, quotes, and mini-essays. The blogs are based on the latest research. Some have been revised and updated for this book. The personal essays are seeing the light of day for the first time; they reflect my own experiences and personality, revealing my quirks, preferences, joys, sorrows, and complaints. I hope they are not TMI—"too much information." But sometimes it's reassuring, or at least interesting, to know what someone else is thinking and doing on this adventure called "aging."

In addition to the essays and personal stories, you'll find these features:

- "One Small Spark:" These random mini-essays, stories, quotes, bits of juicy information, and advice are scattered throughout the text.
- References: Footnotes are found at the end of each essay, highlighted in gray. If you want to fact-check me, I've made it easy for you. If you want to skip over these references, that's fine, too.
- "Other Voices:" I've assembled an array of quotes that will appear after each section or theme. Here you'll find a variety of viewpoints. I hope you find these quotations inspiring, thought-provoking, or just plain funny.

Full disclosure: I am now 75 and enjoying life more than ever, despite an ever-increasing array of annoying, painful, or inconvenient health issues. I would like to pass on the secrets I have learned. My fondest hope is that this book will "spark" your desire to create a happier, healthier life for yourself as you age.

—Meg Rashbaum Selig, August 2020

"Trust your happiness and the richness of your life at this moment. It is as true and as much yours as anything else that ever happened to you."

—Katherine Anne Porter

PART I
OLDER AND HAPPIER

CHAPTER 1

OLDER AND HAPPIER? 5 AMAZING FINDINGS FROM RECENT RESEARCH

It's true: Surveys show that older people are happier people.

I celebrated a big birthday recently. I won't say *which* birthday, but let's just say it was big enough that from now on I'm going to think twice before I buy anything in quantity. Keeping up with the latest research on how to age happily and healthily has become of even more vital personal interest to me than it already was.

When I think of "old age," my mind focuses first on a host of possible ills, from inconveniences like an achy back to serious diseases and disabilities, not to mention the looming "Big D" out there. But much as I like to whine about getting older, I must say I am far happier than at any other point in my life. So I've been wondering: Am I an oddity or do other people feel happier as they enter the "golden years," too? And, if not, is there anything they can do about it?

Fortunately, my personal experience appears to reflect a general pattern. Here are five recent studies that provide fascinating glimpses into the cozy relationship between aging and happiness. Use the specific happiness tips at the end of each study to raise your odds of contentment as you age.

1. In general, surveys show that older people are happier people.

Polls of people at different ages in 149 countries reveal a startling pattern. When asked to rate their life satisfaction on a scale of 1 to 10, most adults in their early 20s reported fairly high happiness levels, with a gradual fall-off as they approached midlife. Adults reported being *least* happy in mid-life, roughly between the ages of 39 and 57, with the happiness low point at age 50.

Here's the most surprising part: As they aged, older adults rated their life satisfaction progressively higher, with happiness ratings rising gradually and steadily from age 50 through the decade of the 90s. Researchers call this process the "U-curve" of happiness. When put on a graph, the results actually form a lop-sided smile.

The data leave room for a variety of interpretations. Maybe knowing our days are numbered helps us savor them even more. But whatever the explanation, health writer Jonathan Rauch asserts that "... studies show quite strongly that people's satisfaction with their life increases, on average, from their early 50s on through their 60s and 70s and even beyond—for many until disability and final illness exact their toll toward the very end."

Exact their toll. Old age certainly is not all sweetness and light. But this counter-intuitive survey research gives cause for optimism. If we do feel happier past age 50 and beyond, then it makes sense to stay healthy so we can enjoy our older years. There's truth in the old saying, attributed to composer Eubie

Blake: "If I'd known I was going to live this long, I'd have taken better care of myself."

So the first step is...live long enough to get old.

If you aren't happy, just wait a few years. You'll be happier!

What you can do: If you aren't happy, just wait a few years. You'll be happier! Meanwhile, take good care of yourself.

2. Older people find happiness in the "ordinary" things.

Young people seek extraordinary experiences—experiences that are novel, exciting, and provide bragging rights. By contrast, older people can find happiness in the so-called ordinary experiences of life—familiar, peaceful, and predictable events. Seniors tend to stop pining for that fabulous trip to the temples of Cambodia and enjoy the small pleasures of a meal at a new restaurant or a visit from a friend.

Of course, this generalization does not apply to everyone. Think of President George H.W. Bush, who famously celebrated his 90th birthday by skydiving out of a plane. Nonetheless, as a general rule, older adults find themselves increasingly delighted by daily-life experiences.

It's encouraging that even with limited finances or impaired health, our waning days can be filled with happy moments.

What you can do: Learn to savor the small moments of your day. Remember that happiness is an "inside job."

3. Meaningful relationships, even online relationships, add to happiness among the aging.

Psychologist Laura Carstensen and her colleagues write: "As people age and time horizons grow short, people invest in what is most important, typically meaningful relationships, and derive increasingly greater satisfaction from these investments." In line with this observation, research suggests that even online connections can lower the risk of depression in retired people by as much as one third compared to those who do not go online.

What you can do: Cultivate relationships that matter. Send cards and emails, make calls, and arrange get-togethers. Join a social media site.

4. Volunteering is a pathway to happiness for many older adults.

People like to feel useful. That's why two-three hours per week of volunteering can bring a host of happiness and health benefits in its wake (more than that has no additional benefit). After examining 73 studies on aging, researchers concluded that volunteering was associated with a lower risk of depression and a stronger feeling of well-being among people 50 and older. They also found health benefits such as greater longevity and better overall health. People who volunteer also developed new relationships, itself a predictor of happiness in older-aged people (see #3 above).

What you can do: Decide on a type of volunteering that fits your personality and values. If you dread your volunteer work, you've made the wrong choice. Choose again! If you don't want a volunteer job, think about friends or family who could benefit from your help or attention. Or, if you love your profession, just keep working.

5. Decide on a purpose for your golden years.

Some elders experience a decline in their sense of purpose in life as they age, but this feeling is by no means inevitable. Protective factors against feelings of isolation and loss of meaning can include volunteer work, frequent contact with family, and continued employment, among others. "Purpose" may even be protective of your brain health, according to *Psychology Today* blogger Maclin Stanley. He cites research that indicates that "people who have a greater sense of purpose in life are more likely to have slower rates of mental decline, even as plaques and tangles develop in their brains. Purpose has also been linked to decreased mortality and happiness in old age."

In fact, setting and reaching achievable and worthwhile goals leads to happiness, whatever your age.

What you can do: Decide on a "purpose project." Your project could range from writing your memoirs for your grandchildren to a social action project. Or, if your purpose in retirement is to have more fun, do that! My wonderful, people-loving aunt enjoyed herself until her last day of life at age 95, when she told the hospice nurse to call her lady friends and cancel her bridge game. Because my aunt loved fun, she invigorated everyone around her. The gift of fun is priceless.

As I re-read these words, I still find it hard to believe that there's such a strong correlation between aging and happiness—even though it's true of me. Old stereotypes—and stereotypes about the old—die hard. But the truth is more complex—and more hopeful. It's reassuring to know that our odds of happiness may actually increase as we age.

© Meg Selig. Posted Jan. 7, 2015, psychologytoday.com.

References

Lop-sided smile. Rauch, J. "The Real Roots of Midlife Crisis," *The Atlantic*, Dec. 2014.

Dean, J. (2014) "Get Your Elders Online for their Mental Health," PsyBlog.com.

"Evidence mounting that older adults who volunteer are happier, healthier." *ScienceDaily.com* (2014). *https://www.sciencedaily.com/releases/2014/08/140829135448.htm*

Stanley, M. (2014) "The Pernicious Decline of Purpose in Life with Old Age," psychologytoday.com.

Goals and happiness. Selig, M. (2009) *Changepower! 37 Secrets to Habit Change Success* (NY: Routledge), p. 222.

Carstensen, L. (2011). *A Long Bright Future.* NY: Broadway Books.

CHAPTER 2

HAPPIER BUT LESS CONFIDENT? WHY OLDER PEOPLE LOSE SELF-ESTEEM... AND HOW TO REGAIN IT

The deplorable reason why older people have lower self-esteem...and how they can regain it.

Research on the relationship between happiness and aging is solid and deep, with all studies pointing to the same conclusion: *Older people are happier people, even when they are coping with problems of declining health and relationship loss.*

Still, there is a disturbing note. A large 2010 study published by the American Psychological Association examined the self-esteem of 3,617 Americans ages 25 to 104 every four years for sixteen years. The conclusion of the researchers was that self-esteem rose steadily until retirement, or about age 60-65, then declined steadily after that.

I was shocked when I came across this study. I could hardly believe it. Wasn't self-esteem the first cousin of happiness? Could you really have one without the other? I was especially bewildered because my own self-esteem, happiness, and age have all risen together. I re-read the study to make sure I understood. Yes, according to the research, self-esteem—the feeling of one's overall worth as a person—did decline later in life.

Offering a shred of optimism, the authors put forth two factors that seemed to staunch the ebb tide of declining self-esteem: "wealth" and/or "health." They speculated that wealth and health might be linked to a greater sense of independence which, in turn, would bolster self-esteem. Or wealth/health might enable an individual to make greater contributions to one's family and society, an action that could also shore up self-esteem. I found these theories disturbing. Could someone really buy their way to self-esteem?

Other studies challenge the idea that there is a steep decline in self-esteem as people age. For example, a study of 462 people, aged 70-103, found that the amount of the decline was minor and occurred chiefly among the oldest-old and those close to death. Self-esteem remained relatively stable in late life, according to this study from 2015. This group of researchers found that four factors helped buttress self-esteem among the elderly: health, cognitive ability, a sense of control, and social inclusion.

Wealth, health, faith in one's cognitive abilities, a sense of control, and relationships—it makes sense that these factors might play a role in maintaining the self-esteem of older people.

The Real Culprit?

However, I suspect that another factor might be a key contributor to the lack of self-esteem among older people: *ageism*. By "ageism,"* I mean both the belief that older people are less important simply because of their age and the widespread discriminatory practices that result from this belief.

Many, if not most, older people have no doubt internalized the ageism of our culture (I am no exception). This internalized ageism cannot help but affect feelings of self-worth. The sense of being "less than" younger or middle-aged people poses a danger to the confidence of any older person, regardless of skills, health, or wealth.

There is fascinating research showing the harmful effects of age stereotyping. In one study, Yale researcher Becca Levy flashed words positively or negatively associated with aging on a screen where they were "seen" only subliminally by older research subjects. "The experiments demonstrated that older people exposed to positive messages about late life showed better recall and more confidence in their abilities than those exposed to negative ones," summarizes Ashton Applewhite, author of *This Chair Rocks: A Manifesto Against Ageism*. (Similar experiments show the effects of "stereotype threats" on Blacks, women, and other stigmatized groups.)

What Does Ageism Look Like?

Here are just a few ways in which ageism might affect the self-esteem of older people:

1. **Employment discrimination.** Job discrimination affects both wealth and self-sufficiency. "How are older people supposed to remain self-sufficient if they're forced out of the job market?" asks Applewhite.

2. **Stereotyping.** Older people are characterized as "geezers," "crones," "senile," and worse. These stereotypes reinforce shame and self-loathing. "Shame can damage self-esteem and quality of life as much as externally imposed stereotyping," according to Applewhite.

3. **Disability discrimination.** People with disabilities are stigmatized in our society; aging adults whose

bodies are failing and must use canes, walkers, and wheelchairs become subject to this set of prejudices in addition to common aging biases.

4. **Dependence discrimination.** Older people often can benefit from help from their children, nursing aides, or spouse. But in our society, it is hard to ask for help because "needing help" is not part of the John Wayne/ total self-reliance ethos. However, the lives of "old- ers"** can narrow significantly if they don't find a way to fight this bias and accept the need for assistance with dignity and creativity.

5. **Judgment about appearance.** "Looking old" is con- sidered a betrayal of our cultural standards of beauty. Women are judged even more harshly than men for the terrible crime of aging. By the way, I am not judging anyone who tries to look younger either. Who could blame anyone for trying to escape society's biased opinions? Or for lifting their own morale by looking better? And some people need to maintain a youthful appearance to stay employed.

What You Can Do

If you are getting older—and you are—and you find yourself feeling "less than" others, begin asking *why*. It could be the ageism in our society, internalized ageism, or a combination of the two.

To make life better for yourself and everyone else, you may want to become an anti-ageism activist. A few potential issues to address: fix the problem of poor compensation and benefits for caregivers of the elderly, campaign against job discrimination, advocate for universal design and other workplace accommo- dations, lobby Medicare to add long-term care and hearing aids benefits, support the expansion of Social Security, work towards absentee voting… and the list could go on.

On the personal level, awareness of internalized ageism can help you see the world and yourself with new eyes. At the very least, you can train yourself to pause and self-correct when you start to feel less deserving of your own respect. You can replace self-stereotyping with the determination to love yourself, respect yourself, and express yourself. Appreciating and valuing who you are is a cornerstone of happiness at any age. And for instant self-esteem, try the three-minute confidence exercise in the next chapter.

If older people themselves can become less ageist, then it is my hopeful guess that future studies about aging and confidence might show a distinct rise in self-esteem among the over-65 group.

© Meg Selig. Posted Jul 05, 2020 on psychologytoday.com.

*The formal definition of ageism, according to Ashton Applewhite, is: "discrimination and stereotyping on the basis of a person's age."

**The wonderful term "olders" was coined by Ashton Applewhite in her book, *This Chair Rocks*.

References

Applewhite, A. (2016). *This Chair Rocks: A Manifesto Against Ageism*. NY: Celadon Books.

"Self-esteem Declines Sharply Among Older Adults While Middle-Aged Are Most Confident," APA, 2010: https://www.apa.org/news/press/releases/2010/04/self-esteem. Original article: Orth, U. et al, "Self-Esteem Development from Young Adulthood to Old Age: A Cohort-Sequential Longitudinal Study," *Journal of Personality and Social Psychology*, 2010, Vol. 98, No. 4, 645– 658.

A study of 462 people. "Self-Esteem is Relatively Stable Late in Life: The Role of Resources in the Health, Self-Regulation, and Social Domains," Wagner, J. et al. *Developmental Psychology*. 2015 Jan; 51(1): 136–149. https://www.ncbi.nlm.nih.gov/pmc/articles/PMC4397980/

Wykle, M.L. et al, eds. *Successful Aging Through the Life Span* (2005). NY: Springer Publishing Co, 108, 153.

One Small Spark:

Age Pride

After I wrote the blog above, I made the decision to cultivate more "age pride." I was soon to be tested.

During a Facetime call, my four-and-a-half-year-old granddaughter wanted to know how old I was. Together we counted to 75. Afterwards she exclaimed, "NanNan, you are old!"

"Yes, I am," I replied, infusing my voice with all the pride I could muster. "Isn't it wonderful that I've lived for so many, many years?"

Silence. Maybe she was absorbing that idea. Maybe I planted a seed.

CHAPTER 3

HOW TO BECOME MORE SELF-CONFIDENT IN THREE MINUTES A DAY

Note: I was so shocked to discover that older people were happier but less self-confident that I decided to include the following blog, one of my all-time favorites. As a result of practicing this exercise, I can truthfully say that I feel more self-confident now, at age 75, than at any other time in my life. May it help you, too! M.S.

The Mystery of Self-Confidence

If you suffer from a lack of self-confidence, you know that it truly is a kind of suffering. You may feel less important than others, unsure of what you think and believe, or unaware of your own strengths. These feelings may cause you to approach life with timidity, defensiveness, or an excessive need to please others.

Some people can project confidence without really owning it, but the kind of self-esteem that is important is not just an act. It is a positive feeling about yourself, your ideas, and your worth that enables you to take good care of yourself, stand on equal footing with others, and feel pride about yourself and how you live your life. (Note: For the purposes of this essay, I am lumping "self-confidence" and "self-esteem" together, though distinctions are sometimes made between them.)

Not all self-confidence is under your control. In fact, by some estimates, about 50% of self-confidence is genetic. Fortunately, you've got the other 50% to work with.

When you use the method described below, you will gradually acquire more inner confidence along with the ability to take actions that will improve your life. You can do this fun mental exercise by yourself, privately, and in very little time.

The Process

The easy exercise for confidence-building is a Daily Success Review. It is a cousin to the famous gratitude exercise, Three Good Things, in which you take some time at the end of the day to focus on three good things that happened to you that day and why. In this variation, you will focus on three successes, large or small, that you had on a particular day.

The process is straightforward: Take three minutes or less to make a mental note of (or write down) one to three successes of your day.

By "successes," I do not necessarily mean major achievements, although if you have them, by all means, bask in their glory. But don't overlook the power of your everyday "small wins." By deliberately focusing on daily victories, you will reinforce your constructive actions and thoughts, thus making it likely you'll have more small wins on subsequent days.

Some of you may be thinking, "Successes?! I don't have successes. My life is a mess." I suspect that many people may not realize all the possibilities there are to feel good about themselves on a given day. So, just to give you some ideas, here are 25 possible small wins to notice as you go through your day:

1. You made a good decision.

2. You took the time to exercise.

3. You felt compassion for yourself when you made a mistake instead of beating yourself up.

4. You responded to a situation in a better way than you normally would.

5. You took a break when you got tired instead of pushing yourself in an unhealthy way.

6. You refrained from making a bad situation worse.

7. You helped someone.

8. You refrained from helping someone because you needed to focus on your own projects.

9. You completed or made progress on a project.

10. You decided that something was not worth doing and quit doing it.

11. You persisted with a task, even when it was unpleasant.

12. You did something healthy for your mind, such as meditating for a few minutes when under stress or... doing the Daily Success Review!

13. You were able to find just the right thing to say to a family member, friend, or colleague.

14. You made a mistake and learned from it.

15. You made a mistake and didn't let it ruin your day.

16. You took the initiative to set up a social occasion or strengthen a friendship.

17. You said no to unreasonable demands or set a boundary that needed to be set.

18. You apologized when you did something wrong and didn't apologize when you didn't.

19. You lived up to your values, even though it was difficult.

20. You set goals for your day and adjusted them when necessary.

21. You got an idea about how to move your life forward in some way.

22. You got an idea about your next work project.

23. You prepared for an event ahead of time so you wouldn't have to rush the next day.

24. You accepted the reality that something couldn't be changed, thus conserving your energy.

25. You paused and reflected on something before you acted, instead of reacting impulsively.

Of course, there is an infinite number of things you might feel good about on a given day. The list above is meant only to give you ideas. With or without the list, can you think of three successes you've already had today?

To see if a Daily Success Review will work for you, try it for a few weeks. Feel free to skip it sometimes, just to keep it fresh. Your goal is to develop a small-success mindset so that you are on the lookout for the many positive things you do as well as the courage you show when you learn from mistakes.

After doing a Daily Success Review on a regular basis, you may learn to recognize a small success immediately after it occurs. When you notice a little victory, you could give yourself an inner compliment, using self-talk like this:

- Hey, I handled that pretty well!"

- "Good decision!"
- "Way to go! You kept your cool under pressure!"

It Should Be Easy

Remember the small wins!

If you can't seem to find successes in your day, you may be searching too hard for extraordinary and dramatic achievements. Remember the small wins!

Teresa Amabile, a professor at Harvard Business School, has researched small wins and their power to build self-confidence. Leah Fessler, writing in *The New York Times,* summarizes Amabile's work this way: "Ms. Amabile's research suggests… that small wins can have just as positive an influence on our sense of self-efficacy, happiness and, ultimately, our productivity as enormous accomplishments do."

Given our brain's negativity bias—the built-in tendency to notice negative things in the environment for the sake of survival, you may also find yourself focusing too much on failures. Of course you can learn from failures, setbacks, and negative events as well as from successes. If you decide to review one of these, give yourself credit. It's not easy to take a hard look at our personal flops. And if the whole day was one mishap after another, just forgive yourself and move on.

Building self-confidence is a process, not an event. But if you've tried this exercise for a few weeks and you still find it difficult to notice your good qualities and actions, you may want to see a therapist for help.

Other Benefits of Focusing on Successes

A Daily Success Review is a great way to know yourself. As you do it, you will begin to see patterns in your successes. You could realize that you have a strength in one area and a weakness in another. You may realize that your passions lie this way not that way. You could notice what you value. You might more easily recognize people, places, and things that lift you up, and people, places, and things that it might be better to avoid.

Just thinking about past successes and values has surprisingly positive effects on behavior, thinking, academic performance, and even IQ. Dr. Jeremy Dean cites research that suggests that recognizing your own successes can raise your IQ about 10 points. Similar types of self-affirmation were shown in other research to increase the test scores of often-marginalized students such as Blacks and female math students.

In a nutshell, being able to savor your successes will make your life more pleasant and more meaningful. Since pleasure and meaning are two essential ingredients of happiness, you will feel happier, too.

Yes, your daily successes may seem small, but often small victories are the sweetest. And maybe those positive actions you took are not so small after all.

© Meg Selig. Posted May 02, 2018, psychologytoday.com.

References

Dean, J. "A Quick and Easy Way to Boost IQ 10%," PsyBlog, April 2018: https://www.spring.org.uk/2018/04/boost-iq.php

Selig, M. "The Amazing Power of 'Small Wins," psychologytoday.com: July 2012: https://www.psychologytoday.com/us/blog/changepower/201207/the-amazing-power-small-wins

Contie, Vicki, "Gene Linked to Optimism and Self-Esteem," NIH: Sept. 26, 2011.

Fessler, L. "Smarter Living: The Power of Low-Stakes Productivity." *The New York Times*, 8.17.2020

Kay, K. & Shipman, C. (2014). *The Confidence Code*. NY: HarperCollins

CHAPTER 4

YOUR PSYCHOLOGICAL PORTFOLIO FOR HEALTHY AGING

"People over the age of 65 have the most stable and optimistic outlook of all adults."
— Laura Carstensen

Because many people think of old age as a bleak time of life, it can be hard to wrap your mind around the idea that the later years really are the "golden years." As aging expert Laura Carstensen writes, "Research shows over and over that most older people are happier than the twenty-somethings who are assumed to be in the prime of life. People over the age of 65 have the most stable and optimistic outlook of all adults."

But there is no doubt that getting older also brings difficult choices and challenges. What mental attitudes can help you navigate the typical transitions of aging and weather the inevitable losses that accompany getting older?

Your Psychological Portfolio

Counseling psychologist Nancy Schlossberg describes three key psychological resources, or "mindsets," that must be cultivated and reshaped as you move into the retirement years. They are:

- Identity
- Relationships
- Purpose

In her book *Revitalizing Retirement*, she calls these resources your "psychological portfolio."

Your psychological portfolio. What a great way to think about all the helpful attitudes and mental habits you've accumulated over a lifetime! In this essay, I'll suggest ways to beef up that psychological portfolio. Along with identity, relationships, and purpose, I'll describe one more resource that can bolster the three others as well as provide satisfaction on its own: the *self-care* mindset.

Knowing your identity and purpose, valuing your key relationships, and staying strong with self-care are important at any age. For "olders,"* these mindsets can assume special prominence when enormous changes in work life, such as retirement, and personal life, such as the death of a spouse, can occur all at once.

Moreover, cultivating these mindsets takes place as older people face the end of life. This literal "deadline" means that spending time in ways that bring meaning, fulfillment, and pleasure becomes more important than ever. ("Death awareness" can be a great motivator and could almost be considered a necessary mindset in itself.)

Here are details about the four mindsets, along with suggestions for strengthening them.

Identity

Your identity is who you are—your evolving sense of self that you carry with you always. Schlossberg further describes it as "what you do, your personality characteristics, and even how you see the world."

Like many people in our society, you may find that your sense of self is tightly connected to your work identity. Who are you if you are not a "doctor, lawyer, merchant, chief?" If retired, how do you respond when others ask, "And what do you do?"

Here are a few suggestions:

1. Don't retire. If you love your work, keep working. As Margaret Mead said, "Sooner or later I'm going to die, but I'm not going to retire."

2. Build your new identity on hobbies and healthy pleasures rather than on work.

3. Formulate a retirement "elevator message." The brief message could include what you did before, what you do now, and your plans for the future.

4. Proudly announce your new roles, for example, your role as a grandparent or volunteer.

5. Recall childhood dreams, and figure out how you still might fulfill them, even in some small way.

6. See a career counselor, coach, therapist, or someone who specializes in retirement issues. Such people can often discern your "superpowers."

7. Find a new career, your "third act." Set up "information interviews" with people who are doing what you might like to do, whether that's volunteer work or paid work.

Relationships

An acquaintance once remarked to my friend Susan** that she was lucky to have such wonderful and enduring friendships. She replied, "Luck has nothing to do with it."

In other words, if you want good relationships, you need to make a deliberate decision to reach out to others and connect in some way—whether in person, via greeting cards, or with video calls.

Strong relationships bolster mental and physical health at any age. Some researchers even find that healthy relationships might be the single most important predictor of happiness in older ages.

These suggestions could give you ideas:

1. Take communication skills classes.

2. Cultivate positive emotions. Such emotions as gratitude, hope, appreciation, and empathy will keep you attuned to "the sunny side of life."

3. Create new communities, actual or online, to substitute for your former work communities. I was glad to see that Schlossberg included coffee groups as a possible community, since my partner has expanded his social circle in this very way. Other support groups might include writers' groups, birthday groups, gardening groups, and political groups.

4. Appreciate your family and strengthen family ties. As friends go off in different directions, your family may assume more importance than ever. Apps such as FaceTime and Zoom make regular family "visits" easy and rewarding.

5. Support your partner's dreams and vice versa. This suggestion by Schlossberg is too often forgotten. You and your significant other can become a "mutual admiration society."

Purpose

More and more research points to a sense of purpose as a key ingredient of a happy, fulfilling life for older people. The amazing physical and psychological benefits include a lower risk of premature death, healthier habits, higher levels of happiness, better sleep, and less loneliness.

Your purpose and your identity are closely linked. Ideally, a purpose project will express some of your most cherished values and goals. (More details in the chapter, "Nine Ways to Find Purpose As You Age.")

To clarify your purpose, try these suggestions, many from Schlossberg's work:

1. Analyze your regrets and figure out a way to bring those missing pieces into your life.

2. Decide your focus. Are you drawn to creativity, leadership, service, working, family, learning, or leisure? I'm always glad to see a goal like "leisure" on someone's list, because not everyone has to have a high-sounding purpose project. A former colleague's motto for retirement is: "If it's not fun, I don't do it."

3. Become a caregiver. Often this role is a necessity, not an option. But many find that taking care of spouse, grandchildren, or friends in need is fulfilling work in itself, especially if you balance it with self-care and other activities that bolster your own identity.

4. Brainstorm and write down as many activities, small or large, that you might enjoy, and star the top three. Does this give you any ideas?

Self-Care

To act on your decisions about identity, purpose, and relationships, you need physical and mental strength. That's why devoting time to appreciating and taking care of yourself is essential. In fact, as you age, having a positive relationship with yourself can be just as important as having a positive relationship with others. A few ideas:

1. Practice self-compassion and kind self-talk. If you feel guilty or ashamed about a time when you were not your best self, use self-compassion to put your actions into better perspective. Possible self-talk: "I was going through a hard time back then." "That was something I needed to work on, and I did." "I did the best I could do with a hard situation."

2. Exercise. I preach the gospel of exercise because it strengthens your body, invigorates your mind, and uplifts your spirits, among many, many other benefits.

3. Rest, relax, and get 7-9 hours of sleep a night. Build these three restorative practices into your life.

4. Build self-confidence. Taking time to notice and savor the positive things you do for yourself and others every day will build self-esteem. I refer not to grand successes but to the small successes you might not notice without a little mindfulness. (Try the "Daily Success Review" in Chapter 3.)

Summary

How will you reshape your identity, purpose, relationships, and self-care program in the last three decades of your life? Make a deliberate decision to improve your "psychological portfolio." Then make a plan. A specific plan will highlight your path to a happier future—at any age.

*The wonderful term "olders" was coined by Ashton Applewhite in her book, *This Chair Rocks*.

**"Susan" refers to my longtime friend, Susan Waugh. Thanks, Susan!

© Meg Selig. Posted Jun 19, 2020, on psychologytoday.com.

References

Schlossberg, N. (2010). *Revitalizing Retirement: Reshaping Your Identity, Relationships, and Purpose*. APA: Washington, D.C.

Carstensen, L. (2011). *A Long Bright Future*. NY: Broadway Books.

CHAPTER 5

12 SIMPLE STEPS TO BEING LESS MISERABLE...AND EVEN HAPPIER

Even in tough times, these 12 strategies will bring a little extra joy to your heart.

Are you waiting until your life is problem-free to be happy? If so, you could be waiting for a long time—like forever.

It's common for all of us to tell ourselves during times of stress, "When I finally have _____ (fill in the blank), or when _____ (fill in the blank) is over, then I can be happy." That first blank could be "more friends," "a committed relationship," or "a better job." The second blank could be anything from "the home repair," "the illness," "she stops drinking," or just a particularly busy time.

But the idea that you can't be happy unless and until some condition is met can itself be a huge barrier to happiness. While it is certainly normal to wish that a period of unusual stress would be over, you could be losing a lot of your precious life by giving in to excessive misery and unhappiness. (I would like to clarify that I am talking here about the relatively predictable crises of everyday life, not catastrophic events. Dealing with trauma is a different process from dealing with stress.)

I'm not suggesting that you fake-happy your way through the day. Within your challenging context, I'm suggesting that you find real happiness, if only for a few minutes at a time. (Of course, if you are feeling depressed, out of control, traumatized, or suicidal, please seek help.)

As you know, older adults are experts at figuring out how to be happy. But everyone could use a refresher course from time to time. Here are a dozen techniques that work for people of all ages. Try a few right now:

1. Slap a label on your negative feelings. Research indicates that labeling your negative feelings will, strangely enough, increase your well-being. Telling yourself, "I'm disappointed" or "I'm angry" or even saying just one feeling word—"resentful," "sad," "frightened"—will ease stress.

It seems odd. Why would labeling your feelings ease stress and unhappiness? Research shows that labeling negative feelings shifts your focus from the "fight-or-flight" part of your brain—the amygdala—to the thinking part of your brain—the prefrontal cortex. Once your "thinker" is on board, you can put your feelings in perspective. I'm always amazed at how well and how fast this "labeling technique" can help me get a grip.

2. Offer yourself some compassion. Talking kindly to yourself could bring moments of comfort. You may not have many people in your life right now who can give you the deep empathy that you need, but you do have one person—you. Refuse to listen to your harsh inner critic.

3. Give yourself permission to be happy even when you are experiencing loss, illness, or other difficulties. Tell yourself that you don't need to feel guilty for wanting moments of relief, happiness, and joy in your life. Then you can...

4. Experience pleasing and healthy distractions. Once you give yourself permission to be happy, you can better allow yourself the experience of small pleasures—a walk, a cup of coffee, a chat with a friend, a visit to the park. Music, books, and films can provide both escape and contentment. Remind yourself that it's OK to have fun, even though part of your life may be falling apart.

5. Hold tightly to your self-care program. Or start one if you don't already have one. Exercise, eat right, connect with friends, and get plenty of sleep. Resist the "false friends" of over-drinking, over-eating, and the couch-potato life.

6. Seek out creative and meaningful activities. Pour your feelings into a hobby or a creative activity. Writing in your journal can help you focus and may even be therapeutic, according to studies by psychologist James Pennebaker and others.

7. Compartmentalize. If the source of your unhappiness is work, put your work struggles in the "work compartment" of your brain. Leave them there when you're at home so you can enjoy your home life. When you get back to work, take those work issues out again, and deal with them as best you can. Taking a mental break from your troubles may even help you envision new solutions.

8. Realize that everything changes. Events change, feelings change. However you feel now, you are likely to feel differently in the future, perhaps even in the next moment. Let "this too shall pass" become your motto.

9. Change one small aspect of your situation. Is there a way to make even a tiny change that will improve your life? "Do one thing different," as therapist Bill O'Hanlon wrote in his book of the same name. Then take another action that will help you. And another.

10. Ask for help. You may think you are admitting defeat by asking for help. Reframe this destructive idea. Instead, think of yourself as the CEO of your own life (because you are), and delegate some responsibilities to others. Don't try to do that home repair yourself—get off that ladder!—and hire someone instead if you can. Use the time you gain for self-care, fun, and meaningful activities. Find a therapist who can be your ally and sounding board.

11. Help others. While it may sound odd to seek to help others when you yourself need help, research shows that helping others will make you happier, among other health benefits. You may also realize that your situation could always be worse—because it could. (If you are already a full-time caregiver, helping others may not be the best tactic for you. Focus on self-care instead.)

12. Be grateful for what you can. Gratitude is the cousin of happiness. Think of three things you are grateful for right now. What is the effect on your mindset?

There are times when searching for happiness could be a way to avoid facing serious problems. For example, if you are unhappy because you are in an abusive or life-threatening situation, focusing on moments of happiness could be a way of avoiding direct action. Call a hotline for help, and get out when you can.

Some extraordinary people can find happiness even under the harshest conditions. Such individuals amaze and inspire me. For example, when poet and author Nina Riggs was diagnosed with metastatic breast cancer, she knew she would die and leave her two young sons behind. Before her death at age 39, she was able to tell her husband, "I have to love these days in the same way I love any other."

When you wait for some external event to occur so that you can be happy, you are taking a passive stance toward your own well-being. Remember, you alone have the ultimate responsibility for your own happiness.

© Meg Selig. Posted on psychologytoday.com, Aug 28, 2017.

References

Whiteman, H. "Embracing negative emotions could boost psychological well-being," *Medical News Today,* August 13, 2017.

Pennebaker, JW & Evans, JF (2014). *Expressive Writing.* Idyll Arbor Press.

Newman, J. "I'm Dying Up Here...," *New York Times,* June 16, 2017.

One Small Spark:

How Old Is "Old?"

Erik Erickson, the great developmental psychologist who divided human life into eight "psychosocial stages," delineated only one stage after adulthood: "mature age." Now that life expectancy has expanded so enormously, many psychologists and sociologists divide older adulthood into three subgroups:

(1) "Young-old age"—age 65 to 74.
(2) "Middle-old age"—75 to 84.
(3) "Old-old age"—85 and above.* Sometimes this group is called "the oldest old."

If our society can expand life expectancy still further, these categories will probably change again.

Note: "Middle age" is usually considered to be ages 45-65. If you have just turned 40, you are not old. In fact, you are not even middle-aged!

*This particular set of categories is from:
https://opentextbc.ca/introductiontosociology/chapter/
chapter13-aging-and-the-elderly/*

CHAPTER 6

GATHERING NECTAR: A PERSONAL ESSAY ON BLISS IN YOUNG-OLD AGE

It was an unusual spot for a revelation.

I was sitting in a pub. Although I don't drink, I love a good sports bar with delicious pub food. My longtime romantic partner Brian and I were shoulder to shoulder at a corner table, idly watching a baseball game, holding hands, and sipping coffee while we waited for our lunch. Before us was a floor-to-ceiling antique wooden bar with lovely carvings and other curlicues. The bottles and glasses sparkled in the glints of sunshine coming through the window. Through an open door, I could see the diners at patio tables and hear the hum of voices from inside and out.

Suddenly I was overcome by an intense feeling of bliss. Everything seemed so sweet and beautiful. My eyes filled with tears. It was a feeling beyond happiness.

In a few moments, the feeling had passed, yet a sense of contentment remained. What had happened? I still don't know. Maybe the positive forces in the universe dropped down on me for a few joyous moments. Maybe the combination of loving touch and the anticipation of a good meal filled me with gratitude. Maybe I was coming down with a rare neurological disease. Maybe it was the coffee. Yeah, the coffee.

But as I thought about this incident, I remembered that it was not the first time I had experienced such a moment. A few months before, Brian and I had taken a walk along the Mississippi River on a perfect late summer day. As we strolled, it seemed that every buzzing, flying, and hopping insect had emerged to gather nectar from the flowers along the trail. There were butterflies of all sorts, grasshoppers, bees and other insects, along with soaring and roosting birds, frogs, and even a harmless snake or two, all crossing the trail as we went by. Each one was savoring the last fruits of summer.

Again, I felt a rare ecstasy—a type of aliveness, a feeling of belonging to the community of nature that swirled around us.

Another time Brian and I went to visit relatives in Washington, DC. For years, when my daughter and her family lived there, I had been a regular guest at a small hotel with an excellent restaurant. I had savored numerous breakfasts and dinners there.

We walked to that restaurant from our current hotel. As we entered, I saw that this restaurant was as charming and welcoming as ever. My eyes swam with tears, as if I had encountered a wonderful old friend—which, in a way, I had.

What was happening?

● ● ●

These three incidents all occurred around the time of my 70th birthday. At 70, I felt little different than I had at 40, but it was a Big Number, so big that it was hard to deny that I was—say it!—OLD.

I had kept up with the research on happiness and aging. I'd learned that older people are happier people, despite what younger people might predict.

But my unusual experiences seemed of a different order than mere happiness. I wasn't sure if I was the only one who was visited by moments of bliss in old age or if my experiences were typical. I still haven't found the answer.

But I do have a theory.

• • •

My theory is that by age 70, some of us realize that we have now reached the time of "The September Song." One of the most beautiful songs ever written, the song reflects our poignant knowledge that "the days dwindle down to a precious few." We realize there is an end to our living.

Like the bees and butterflies, we instinctively know that it's time to gather nectar—to savor it, to down it as fast as we can, to appreciate everything, and to feel grateful, even in times of loss. As therapist Mary Pipher writes, "As we walk out of a friend's funeral, we can smell wood smoke in the air and taste snowflakes on our tongues."

Mother Nature is sometimes "red in tooth and claw," but in this case, she is merciful. Yes, we are going to die, but first we get to experience the ecstasy of gathering nectar. Whether felt as sensuous or spiritual or loving, we get to feel the bliss of being alive as we approach Old Age.

© Meg Selig, 2015. Revised 2020.

References

Pipher, M., "The Joy of Being a Woman in Her 70s." New York Times, 1/12/2019.

* "The September Song" was composed by Kurt Weill; the lyrics are by Maxwell Anderson.

OTHER VOICES:
Aging and Happiness

"Aging is an extraordinary process where you become
the person you always should have been."

—David Bowie

"I despair of ever being able to reconcile my overall sense
of well-being, self-confidence, achievement, and pleasure in the
richness of the present with the image I see in the mirror."

—Vivian Sobchack

"In ancient China, the Taoists taught that a constant inner smile,
a smile to oneself, insured health, happiness, and longevity.
Why? Smiling to yourself is like basking in love: you become your
own best friend. Living with an inner smile is to live in harmony
with yourself."

—Mantak Chia

"If there is one thing I've learned in my years on this planet,
it's that the happiest and most fulfilled people are those who
devoted themselves to something bigger and more
profound than merely their own self-interest."

—John Glenn

"Aging is not 'lost youth,' but a new stage of
opportunity and strength."

—Betty Friedan

PART 2
LIVING LONGER

CHAPTER 7

WHAT IS THE ONE ESSENTIAL KEY TO LONG LIFE?

It turns out to be a personality trait rather than a particular behavior. The answer is...

If you desire to live a long, healthy life, you will be interested in the research results described in *The Longevity Project* by Howard S. Friedman and Leslie R. Martin.

According to the authors, there are some things, however valuable in other ways, which do NOT lead to longevity:

- Taking life easy—being carefree. (Carefree people often don't pay attention to health matters.)
- A sociable personality. (Extroverts are more likely to cave in to social pressures to drink and smoke.)
- Cheerfulness and excessive optimism. (Rose-colored glasses make real threats harder to see.)

If *you* were searching for the fountain of youthful old age, where would you look? Friedman and Martin's springboard was an eight-decade study—the Terman study, headed by psychology researcher Lewis Terman in the 1920s. The authors mined mounds of data that had been accumulated from Terman's 1500+ subjects who had been studied from childhood until their death. They also re-analyzed the data using modern research methods and the results of other long-term studies.

So, what was the one factor that turned out to be the main highway to longevity? As an avid reader of health and psychology articles and books, even I was surprised at the answer. It turns out to be a personality trait rather than a particular behavior. Can you guess what it is?

The surprising answer is: **Conscientiousness**. Conscientious people are dependable, hard-working, persistent, and well-organized—even a little obsessive. Amazingly, conscientiousness was the best predictor of longevity when measured in childhood, AND it was the best predictor of longevity when measured in adulthood. As the authors point out, good people DON'T die young, despite what Billy Joel sings in his seductive song. And virtue is not just its own reward—you get long life as well. This is a satisfying result.

Now that I've revealed the answer, it seems so obvious. Of course conscientious people would live longer! As the authors point out, they are more likely to take actions to protect their health, and they engage in fewer risky activities: "They are less likely to smoke, drink to excess, abuse drugs, or drive too fast. They are more likely to wear seat belts and follow doctors' orders." Every day they make decisions that keep them on a healthy life path.

Plus, conscientious people are drawn to other conscientious people. Their personality leads them into healthier relationships and situations, including happier marriages, good friendships, and healthy work situations.

The researchers found other predictors of long life as well. Longevity tends to come to those who:

- Connect with others.
- Associate with healthy people.

- Develop healthy habits.
- Help others.
- Stay physically active throughout life.
- Are moderate worriers, but not catastrophizers.

What does all this mean for you? There are many lessons in *The Longevity Project*, but there's one especially to take to heart. To live a long life, become the kind of conscientious person you would want as your own best friend.

© Meg Selig. Posted March 23, 2011, psychologytoday.com.

References

Friedman, H.S. and Martin, L.R. (2011). *The Longevity Project*. NY: Hudson Street Press.

CHAPTER 8

FOUR MORE SURPRISING SECRETS TO A LONGER LIFE

What you do in your spare time could make a big difference in your life span.

4 Strange Ways to Extend Your Life Expectancy

How could you live a longer, happier, and healthier life? Whatever your age, you have a vested interest in the answer. As a member of the Medicare generation, the question is of vital importance to me. Amazingly, I am enjoying life today more than ever, and that joy motivates me to keep going for as long as possible.

By the way, I am not alone in my late-in-life happiness: Large-scale research studies reveal that older adults experience happier lives as they age, even if they have a few physical ailments. What a surprising and wonderful finding—and I want you to experience this same happiness. So I've scanned for the latest research on extending our lifespan. What's the latest? First, let's take a quick look at what we already know.

Well-Known Longevity Factors

Research has supported the links between longevity and the following behaviors:

- Exercise. Exercise! EXERCISE! Even small doses will extend your life. (By how much? See the next chapter.)
- Good relationships. Surround yourself with caring people.
- Reducing stress. Aim for challenges that stretch you but don't overwhelm you.
- Managing your money wisely. Debt is a willpower vampire, a huge stressor, and a joy-killer. Have a financial cushion.
- Eating healthy foods most of the time.
- Sleeping for 7-8 hours per night.
- Engaging in meaningful activities, having a sense of purpose.
- Drinking coffee. (Oh, joy!)

In their 2011 book, *The Longevity Project*, Howard Friedman and Leslie Martin reported that the most important factor in longevity was not a behavior, per se, but a character trait: conscientiousness. Conscientious people take care of their health, keep their medical appointments, are responsible to friends and family, and practice healthy habits.

And Now… Recent Longevity Studies

Recent research adds four somewhat surprising recommendations to the list:

1. Read more books.

A recent study found that 30 minutes of reading books per day was associated with a two-year increase in life span for those 50 or older. What validation for those of us who love to read anyway! And that's what you are doing at this moment! According to the study:

The research team examined the reading habits of 3,635 people who were 50 or older and their survival was observed over 12 years follow-up. Factors such as education, gender, marital status, wealth, health conditions and depression were controlled for in the study.

Further, the longevity bonus was higher for *book* readers than for magazine and newspaper readers, which, in turn was higher than for non-readers. Book readers who read up to the standard of 30 minutes a day (or 3.5 hours a week) were 17 percent less likely to die over the 12-year follow-up. That's a big bump in life expectancy.

Exactly why book-reading can contribute to a longer life is unclear, even to the study's authors. Obviously, reading would have cognitive benefits. Because book reading keeps you sharper, maybe such readers would take fewer risks that could lead to mortal accidents. Maybe readers are more *introverted*, making them less likely to cave in to social pressures to drink, smoke, or engage in other risky activities. Another possibility: You have to settle down and concentrate in order to read, so could it have some of the calming effects of meditation?

Caution: If you spend too much time on your duff with a book, you will be at higher risk for diabetes, low mood, and weight gain. Remember the cry, "Sitting is the new smoking?" I never believed that sitting was as bad as smoking for your health, but a plethora of research does warn us about the hazards of sitting. So, if you decide to read more, get up every hour and move around for five-ten minutes. Your body and mind will thank you.

Recommendation: Read more *and* move more. If you are like me and can't sit still for more than 50 minutes anyway, you are probably well protected against "sitting diseases."

2. Help others...but don't wear yourself out.

Giving the right dose of emotional support to others will extend your life span. In a study of 500 people over age 70, those who helped out their families and friends by giving occasional support, whether to their children, grandchildren, or even other people's children, reaped the benefit of a longer life.

Cautions: The adage, "Moderation in all things," seemed to apply to this particular helping situation. Too much caregiving can be stressful. For example, in

Know your "Goldilocks point" for helping out—not too much, not too little, but just right.

the study cited above, *custodial* grandparents experienced more stress than those who simply provided occasional physical and emotional support. And high caregiver stress is associated with negative health outcomes. But with too little caregiving, you may be at risk of sinking into isolation or self-absorption.

Recommendation: Know your "Goldilocks point" for helping out—not too much, not too little, but just right. If you sense that you are getting overloaded, cut back on your caregiving.

3. Connect through Facebook...but not too much.

It has long been known that social networks are a strong predictor of longevity. Good relationships buffer us from stress, lowering our risk for illness and early death. But this year, researchers from the University of California at San Diego studied *12 million* (not a misprint) Facebook users and discovered that even *online* relationships are associated with a lower risk of death for those born between 1945 and 1989. Facebook users were about 12 percent less likely to die than those not on Facebook. Of Facebook users, those who lived the longest had these traits:

1. They interacted with others offline, not just on Facebook.

2. Individuals with average or large Facebook networks lived longer than those with smaller ones.

3. Those who accepted the most friendship requests lived longer. (But watch out for scammers.)

By the way, some activities on Facebook were *not* correlated with a longer life, including the number of "likes" your posts received.

Cautions: As people age, some friendships will be lost through geographical distance, death, and divorce. It's comforting to know that online contact with friends could mitigate these harsh realities, as long as face-to-face friendships can also be cultivated. *(Note: There are issues with privacy and the use of your data on any social media site, including Facebook. It should also be noted that Facebook collaborated with this study.)*

4. Enjoy yourself at a museum, a concert, or the theatre.

In a 2019 study cleverly titled, "The Art of Life and Death," British researchers explored whether people aged 50 and older received a longevity benefit from attending arts events. These researchers studied 6710 older people over a 14-year period, correlating the participants' self-reports with death reports from the National Health Service register. The results were astonishing:

- Those who attended arts activities just one-two times per year had a 14% lower risk of dying compared to those who did not.
- Frequent attenders of arts events—an event every few months or so—had a whopping 31% lower risk of dying compared to those who didn't patronize the arts.

These results held true even after the researchers corrected for socioeconomic status, sex, and health factors. I've always said it, and it's true: The arts give life.

In a Nutshell

Read. Help others. Connect via Facebook. Enjoy the arts. These pleasurable activities will improve the moment and deliver on a longer life as well.

© Meg Selig. Posted to psychologytoday.com, Jan. 5, 2017. Revised 2020.

References

Dean, M. "The Right Reading Materials Can Extend Your Life Two Years," http://www.healthiestblog.com/2016/08/reading-longevity.php

"Increased life expectancy among family caregivers," *ScienceDaily*: https://www.sciencedaily.com/releases/2013/10/131015093744.htm

"Life Long and…Facebook?" *ScienceDaily:* https://www.sciencedaily.com/releases/2016/10/161031165135.htm

"The art of life and death: 14 year follow-up analyses of associations between arts engagement and mortality in the English Longitudinal Study of Ageing," BMJ, Dec. 2019.

CHAPTER 9

WHAT IS THE EXACT "DOSE" OF EXERCISE NEEDED FOR LONGEVITY?

Studies reveal the exact daily exercise minutes that add years to your life.

Want to live a long, healthy life? One key is exercise. But how much? Happily, researchers have mined demographic data to unearth the exact "doses" of exercise needed to lengthen your life.

The questions:

These "dose-response" studies provide answers to these questions:

- How many minutes of brisk walking (or any moderate exercise) do you need to do per day to increase your life expectancy?

- If you dislike exercising, what's the very *least* amount you can get away with and still earn a longevity boost?
- For exercise go-getters, what's the amount of brisk walking that provides the *most* extra years of life for your exercise input?

The latest research by expert epidemiologist I-Min Lee of Harvard Medical School and her associates provides the answers. Her work is based on studies of over 650,000 people over 40, followed on average for 10 years.

The answers:

After intense number crunching to control for different variables, the research backs up what we all know intuitively—almost any amount of regular exercise promotes longevity. And even small amounts of exercise can make a big difference.

For example, people who chose to walk briskly for just **11 minutes** per day (75 minutes each week) added 1.8 years to their life, compared to non-exercisers. That's a nice boost for 11 minutes of walking per day. And it gets better. Those who walked **22 minutes** every day (or 150 minutes/week or 30 minutes 5 days a week, following the federal recommendation) gained 3.4 years of life on average.

The people who increased their life span the most walked **43 minutes** a day, lengthening their life by an average of 4.2 years. After 43 minutes, the benefits of exercising tended to level off. (Note to runners and other vigorous exercisers: You received the same benefit, but in about half the time.)

So what's your choice? 11 minutes of moderate exercise/day? 22 minutes? 43 minutes? Pick your pleasure and live a longer life.

Perspective

Naturally, a long life need not be your only reason to exercise regularly. Exercise has numerous other benefits for mind, body, and spirit, as piles of research tells us. And exercise is not the only factor in longevity. Research shows that people who live long lives tend to be responsible and conscientious, engage in fewer risky activities, are non-smokers, and find their way into healthier relationships. They live in an environment with little air pollution or lead pollution and just-right amounts of stress. They inherited good genes from their parents.

While some longevity factors are beyond your control, the choice to exercise for 11 minutes per day—or whatever your chosen exercise level—is a mini-goal that's realistic, specific, and measurable—and that pays off big in the long run.

© Meg Selig. Posted May 09, 2013, psychologytoday.com.

References

A special thanks to Dr. I-Min Lee for clarifying some aspects of her research, found here:

http://www.ncbi.nlm.nih.gov/pmc/articles/PMC3491006/

Air pollution. http://www.hsph.harvard.edu/news/mag-
azine/f12-six-cities-environmental-health-air
-pollution/

One Small Spark:

How to "Spark" an Exercise Habit

If you want to bring regular exercise into your life, start small. Even 10 minutes a day will bring benefits, so don't feel you have to set the bar high.

Here's the **"spark:"** Right after every exercise session, give yourself an inward shout-out. Examples: "Hey, I did it!" "Good for me." "Way to take care of yourself, Self!" "Yes!!" Try these mini-cheers and see what works for you. You could even pat your shoulder or pump your fist. According to habits expert B.J. Fogg, these small "celebrations" will wire your new habit into your brain and make the habit stronger.

CHAPTER 10

"HEALTHSPAN" OR LIFESPAN: HOW TO LIVE SMART AND HEALTHY UNTIL THE END

How could you make your "healthspan" equal to your lifespan?

Lifespan or "Healthspan?"

What if you knew that you were going to live, say, until the age of 90? How much of that time would you like to live in good health?

Most of us would likely shout, "Are you kidding? All of it, of course!"

What you are asking for is the longest "healthspan" possible. "Healthspan" is a word that's been coined relatively recently. "Lifespan" refers to the period between birth and death; "healthspan" is the number of years you live in the best health possible. And if you possess reasonably good health, you will be able to pursue activities that are meaningful and enjoyable to you.

I love the concept of "healthspan." It's a great way to think about what actions your "future self" might appreciate. For example, I've decided that my future self would appreciate frequent visits to my daughter and her family, so my goal is to be fit enough to withstand the rigors of traveling.

What is one thing you could do to extend **your** healthspan? What actions could keep you healthier and stronger, both mentally and physically, until your last days on earth? By the end of this blog, you'll have some ideas for goals that could enrich your life right now while raising your odds for a better future.

Healthspan Heroes

First, a little more about healthspan...

If your healthspan equals your lifespan, you will be healthy and functional up until the moment of death. This is actually possible! For example, the father of a friend, a man in his late 80's, went out one morning to play tennis with his buddies. When he returned, he said, "It was a great game! I feel a little tired though, so I think I'll take a nap." He died during the nap. Then there was my 95-year-old aunt. One day she felt sick. "I'm going to cancel my bridge game," she told her home-health nurse. Then she fell into a coma and died later that day. Her lifespan was only 8 hours longer than her healthspan.

Sadly, these two stories are the exception rather than the rule. Most of us will probably suffer through some period of ill health before we die, hopefully just weeks not years. Some will have chronic illnesses that could greatly impair their functioning. And even if you are a health nut, your life could be disrupted by things that you cannot control—accidents, bad luck, and sudden illness.

But if the Fates are kind, we do have some power to increase our healthspan, making the time between healthy life and death is as short as possible.

Thought Experiment: Healthspan Habit Changes

Here's a little thought experiment that could help you decide on a healthspan resolution. Ask yourself this question: "What activities make life worth living for me right now?" You might come up with 1-4 ideas. Choose one to focus on. Got it? Then fill in the blank below.

For the rest of my life, I would like to be able to _____. To do this, I will need to take at least one of the following action steps:

1.

2.

3.

Choose just one action step to work on right now so you can focus your willpower. If your action step seems too daunting, shrink it into a step that feels easy and doable.

Here are two examples of healthspan goals and action steps:

Healthspan Goal: Stay mentally sharp. Possible action steps:

- Regular aerobic exercise. Research increasingly tells us that exercise protects brain function.
- Learning activities.
- Meaningful activities, like volunteer work or personal projects.

Decide on one option and make a plan to follow through. For example, if you want to exercise more, you could write exercise times in your schedule, aiming eventually for the gold standard of 150 minutes/week. Less than that is fine, too. Just do the best you can.

Healthspan Goal: Maintain friendships/avoid loneliness. Possible mini-goals:

- Call a friend once a week.
- Arrange a get-together with a friend at least once a month.
- Send cards for birthdays and other occasions.

No one is immune to the ups and downs of life. But the good news is that loneliness, disease, and disability are not an inevitable part of aging, especially with a little luck and planning. For a long and happy healthspan, take good care of yourself now. Your future self will thank you.

© Meg Selig. Posted on psychologytoday.com, Dec 28, 2015.

CHAPTER 11
MY LUCKY BREAKS: A PERSONAL ESSAY ON LONGEVITY

I am 75, relatively healthy, and living a good life. Why am I so fortunate? Is it because I am a paragon of good habits like exercising, eating right, and flossing? Partly. I'll take some credit for quitting smoking, maintaining the same weight for 50 years, and exercising almost daily.

Or maybe my happy old age is due to my parents. I was the fortunate daughter of a middle-class family. There was enough money for summer camp and piano lessons, enrichment classes and vacations. My parents were kind, encouraging people, who modeled a healthy lifestyle and generously shared their good genes with me.

As a White person, I was also blessed with numerous invisible privileges. A sense that I had a place at the table. A confidence that I could follow whatever career I wanted. A feeling I could overcome obstacles, even sexism, with the help of other like-minded people. From an early age, the wind was at my back.

But there is yet another reason for my longevity and happiness: Luck. Dumb Luck. Let me explain.

• • •

I fell countless times in my 71st year. I'd fallen before, but it was usually more of an injury to my pride than to my body. My M.O. for handling falls had been to spring up as fast as possible as if to say, "Hey, I'm sure you didn't notice that. I didn't really fall. And even if I did, I'm fine. Just fine."

Falls for older people are often the prelude to broken hips or other broken bones, followed by surgery and a lengthy stay in a rehab facility. The statistics tell us that falling can drastically affect both health and lifespan. Introducing an NPR Health segment, Steve Innskeep intoned ominously: "One of every 5 people who breaks a hip after age 50 dies…within a year. It's not the fall that kills people…it's the complications that come after."

So my falls could have led to disaster or even death.

My first and worst fall occurred at 4 a.m. one dark night. I had an excruciating leg cramp. Rather than stretch it out in the bedroom and possibly wake my partner, I stumbled into the bathroom. I must have slipped on the area rug and lost consciousness because the next thing I knew, I was lying on the tile floor. A quick glance in the mirror revealed a huge knot on my forehead and various purple bruises on my face. I went to the ER where I was given a battery of tests. Verdict: No problems. (Note: Area rugs are a trip hazard! Take them up and/or away!)

And then there were the "minor" falls:

- I fell in the aisle of an airplane, tripping over a metal rug fastener. I grabbed onto a seatback, wrenching my wrist, but was otherwise unharmed.
- I fell on a moving sidewalk in an airport because I was

talking with my daughter and son-in-law and hadn't realized the sidewalk was ending. No wonder they had looks of horror on their faces! How I managed to scramble to my feet after that one, I cannot tell you.

- I fell on the ice in early spring, landing on my rump with a big thud. I landed so hard that I could not immediately get up. By some miracle, I didn't break anything.
- Later that summer, I tripped on a raised part of the sidewalk and fell forward on my hands and knees. Again, I was basically unhurt, even though I had numerous bruises, scrapes, and cuts that required bandaging for over a week.

My misadventures could inspire a Dr. Seuss poem: "I fell in the airport/ I fell on the ice/ I fell on the sidewalk/ It wasn't so nice."

Why did I escape from all these falls relatively unscathed? I like to think that my exercise regimen may have had a protective effect. Maybe it did. And I learned recently that quitting smoking (which I did in my twenties) and taking estrogen* (which I do to this day for bone strength) also reduce the risk of hip fractures.

On the other hand, I've been diagnosed with osteopenia. "Osteopenia" is a common medical condition in which bones thin and weaken. If it worsens, osteopenia can become osteoporosis, which involves even thinner bones and therefore an even higher risk of fracture after falls. It turns out that your bones are densest in your thirties; it's all downhill from there.

So I was lucky. But I knew I had to stop tempting fate and figure out a way to stay upright.

• • •

I'm here to tell you that changing your behavior to avoid falls is possible. Now when I take walks, I pay more attention to my environment instead of getting lost in thought. I've begun consciously lifting my feet higher to avoid raised places in the sidewalk. I never leave for a walk without my phone so I can call home in case of emergency. But it's impossible to be mindful 100% of the time, so I must—again—credit good luck.

"Have you fallen within the past year?" For the last four years, I've been able to proudly answer "no" to this screening question, asked by the medical people at my various doctor's offices.

• • •

Reaching 75 has made me feel humble. I have had plenty of advantages in the game of life. But I know that I'm still in the game because of my lucky breaks. As I look forward and backward, I can only feel grateful for that.

©Meg Selig, 2020.

*Estrogen is not a good choice for every woman. Consult with your doctor about the risks and benefits for you.

OTHER VOICES:
Living Longer

"Atheists have an excellent longevity record because we have no place to go after we die, so we take good care of ourselves and our world while we are here."

—Madalyn Murray O'Hair

"The secret of longevity…is to keep breathing."

—Sophie Tucker

"When asked the recipe for a good old age, I often give a list: good genes, good luck, enough money, and one good kid, usually a daughter."

—Louise Aronson, MD, geriatrician

"Back when I was young, only athletes exercised. We played dodgeball in gym class and did some other silly shit—but if we had known back then that we needed to exercise on a regular basis our entire lives, a whole lot of my friends would probably still be here."

—"Ma," in *It's Not All Downhill from Here,* by Terry McMillan

"Take care of your body as if you were going to live forever; and take care of your soul as if you were going to die tomorrow."

—St. Augustine

PART III
SAFE, HEALTHY, AND WISE

CHAPTER 12

THE BEST BRAIN FOOD MAY NOT BE A FOOD

How can you keep your brain healthy, alert, and functioning optimally for as long as possible?

The Most Important Activity for Brain Health

You, like me, probably want to "drop dead smart," avoiding any adverse events or diseases that could damage your brain. But how can you keep your brain healthy, alert, and functioning optimally until the day you die?

Of course you have to feed your brain with healthy food. That's a given. But the best brain food may not even be a food. Hint: It's an activity.

Is it learning a new language? Doing crossword puzzles? Having a mission in life? Calling a friend? No, although these activities are helpful for mental stimulation, happiness, and a long life, the key to brain health is something else:

Regular exercise.

You already know that regular exercises promotes longevity. In addition, evidence is piling up that mild to moderate aerobic exercise like brisk walking may protect your brain from dementia and from other insults of aging.

The Evidence

Here are summaries of a few recent research studies that link exercise with a healthy brain:

1. **Exercise and memory.** Exercise guru Gretchen Reynolds reported in the *New York Times* that when a group of 120 older men and women followed either a walking program or were part of a control group, the walkers performed better on cognitive tests and regained volume in the hippocampus—a part of the brain responsible for memory, certain types of learning, and the genesis of new brain cells. A typical 65-year-old walker developed the hippocampus of a 63-year-old. (My new goal: A youthful hippocampus.)

2. **Exercise and name/face recognition.** In a study on exercise and memory, researchers compared exercisers to "sitters." First, all participants were given a name-face matching test. After one group exercised for 30 minutes while the other sat quietly, both groups were given a second test. Exercisers improved their scores, while the resting volunteers stayed the same. This boost in short-term memory could come in handy in reducing those embarrassing I-know-I-know-you-but-who-are-you moments.

3. **Activity and cognitive function.** In a large Canadian study of elderly adults, those who were active around the house and garden, took short walks, and cooked maintained their cognitive function for the 2-5 years of the study, whereas the sedentary adults scored

significantly worse on the same tests. Okay, I'm off to do the dishes right now!

4. **Slowing cognitive decline.** Another study, mostly of women in their 70's, showed that cognitive decline slowed significantly in those women who kept active in the same kind of modest way as those in the Canadian study above.

5. **Preventing dementia.** After reviewing 130 papers, scientists from the Mayo Clinic have concluded that exercise that gets your heart pumping (aerobic exercise) may be an important therapy against dementia.

There's lots more evidence based on animal studies, but since I have very few readers who are rodents, I won't cite it here. And, naturally, more research needs to be done with human subjects.

Summing Up

"Brain health" is just one of many reasons to motivate yourself to exercise regularly. Exercise can also: improve your mood; strengthen your bones; boost your immune system; lower your risk for heart disease, diabetes, high blood pressure, and colon cancer; control your weight by making your cells burn extra energy; reduce blood pressure; build muscle mass; help you sleep better; enhance your sex life; and more.

So, as the old song says, "Feed your head!" Just do it with exercise.

© Meg Selig. Posted on psychologytoday.com, July 7, 2012.

References

Exercise and memory smarts. Reynolds, G., "How Exercise Could Lead to a Better Brain," NYT, April 18, 2012.

Name-face recognition. Reynolds, G., "How Exercise Benefits the Brain," NYT, Nov. 30, 2011.

Slowing cognitive decline. Reynolds, G., "How Exercise Can Keep the Brain Fit," NYT, July 27, 2011.

Preventing dementia. "Aerobic exercise may reduce the risk of dementia, researchers say," *ScienceDaily*, Sept. 8, 2011.

CHAPTER 13

7 LESSONS FROM A CROSSWORD PUZZLE

Can doing crossword puzzles prevent mental decline?

Every now and then, an article appears in a respectable publication suggesting that doing crosswords might prevent mental decline in older people. I had always hoped it was true.

Actually, no one knows for sure. Some research says: Crosswords *do* prevent mental decline. Other research says: Crosswords *don't* prevent mental decline. Take your pick!

Since crosswords are a form of mental stimulation, I'm betting they are good for the brain. Of course, I would like to believe this to justify my habit of doing the *New York Times* crossword puzzle every day. Anyway, whatever the data says, just because crosswords are so much fun, I intend to keep at it, one clue at a time. Even if there were no benefits beyond the activity itself, I would still indulge in it. Let's face it, I'm a word nerd.

Whether crosswords are good for your brain or not, this pleasant activity does have other benefits. For example, the practice of doing crosswords can build a set of attitudes useful for coping with life. Here are seven lessons from a crossword puzzle that can enliven your mind and spirit:

1. **Enjoy the flow.** Crosswords put us in a trance state—I call it "Letterland." Psychologists call this state "flow"—a state of being so immersed in what you are doing that the rest of the world falls away. Flow activities, like knitting, sketching, writing, running, or gardening, give your mind a break from boredom, pain, or worry while either doing you no harm or actively doing you good. These activities cost you little and benefit you a lot.

2. **Take a break—the answer will come.** Recent research suggests that taking a break can pump up your creative juices and restore your focus. When it comes to crosswords, taking a short break can restore your brain-power, enabling you to see a mistake or find an answer. It's amazing how solvable a crossword problem can be once you've stepped away from it and returned. For a small, daily "aha" experience, do a crossword.

3. **You'll get better with directed practice.** With practice, you pick up a bit of crosswordese—those dumb words that you only see in puzzles. After a while, certain words become old, quirky friends. You recognize the animals that populate many puzzles—the eels, emus, and ants, for three—or the vowel-laden actors that take their bows again and again—Alda, Uma, and Asner, among others.

4. **Correcting your mistakes can be rewarding.** Making errors in the crossword grid can be frustrating and annoying at first. But the more you do puzzles, the more fun it becomes to track down your errors and correct them. You correct, you learn, you move on.

Psychologists would say you are developing a "growth mindset," the belief that setbacks are just a normal part of learning.

5. **You know more than you think you know.** It's awesome when an answer pops up from somewhere deep in your unconscious. "I didn't even know I knew that!" you think. Sometimes even one letter can poke a neuron embedded deep within your brain and you magically **get it.**

6. **Small steps get a big job done.** At first, a hard puzzle may seem impossible. But word by word, step by step, you fill in the grid and complete the puzzle. Learning to chip away at a crossword is like using small steps to chip away at a big goal. Little by little, you increase your walking program, write a book, or create a garden.

7. **Sometimes you need help.** The *New York Times* Saturday puzzle is usually too challenging for me. My partner and I have created a ritual of passing it back and forth until it's done. Okay, sometimes we cheat and use Google, The Great and Powerful, for an answer. At other times we "go to Rex," solver extraordinaire Rex Parker. Sometimes you need the help of an outside expert to solve a problem. There's no shame in that.

Of course, doing crosswords, like any human activity, can spiral out of control. I once knew someone who avoided his homework by doing puzzle after puzzle after puzzle. For him, crosswords were like those potato chips—"You can't eat just one." But most of us can stop after one crossword. Even if not, I would call crosswords a "positive addiction," somewhat like running.

So, crosswords may or may not keep the brain smart and youthful. I'm sure there will be more research, and I'll be rooting for better cognitive health through crosswords. But whatever the outcome of future studies, I'm sticking with crosswords. I highly recommend the crossword habit. Word by word, you may find yourself learning life lessons that will help you in ways you never anticipated.

© Meg Selig. First posted Feb 21, 2013, on psychologytoday. com. Revised 2020.

References

Adrienne Rafael, "This is your brain on crosswords," March 2020, https://blogs.scientificamerican.com/ observations/this-is-your-brain-on-crosswords/

One Small Spark:

A Riddle

Question: What goes up but never comes down?

Answer: Your age.

From "Garfield," by Jim Davis.

CHAPTER 14

12 QUICK MINI-MEDITATIONS TO CALM YOUR MIND AND BODY

These 30-second meditations are invisible, fun, and surprisingly effective.

Could I have 30 seconds of your time? OK. Now try this: Sit or stand up straight in a comfortable position. Breathe in, breathe out. Pause. One more time, this time a little slower and deeper: Breathe in, breathe out. Now, one more time: Breathe in, breathe out.

Do you feel a bit less stressed? Probably so. That's because you just did a *mini-meditation* called "Three-Breath Practice." (Actually, I find that even "One-Breath Practice" can be helpful.)

No Time, No Desire to Meditate? No Problem!

When we think of meditation, we usually think of a **formal meditation**, in which the meditator sits quietly for a designated amount of time, say 20-40 minutes, focusing on the breath or another object of contemplation. In **mindfulness meditation**, when upsetting thoughts, sensations, or feelings interfere, as they always do, experienced meditators learn to notice them, let them pass by, and then return to paying attention to the breath.

Evidence for the benefits of mindfulness meditation continues to pile up. Numerous studies suggest that meditating can improve heart health and mental health, boost immune response, lower stress, decrease blood pressure, improve healthy aging of cells, and much more. In fact, a recent study indicated that meditation could be just as beneficial as a *vacation*, but with longer-lasting effects.

I don't plan to give up vacations any time soon. But the more I read such studies, the more determined I become to establish a stronger meditation practice. I want those benefits! But then I remember that I don't really *like* long meditations. In fact, I've dropped in and dropped out of the meditation habit numerous times. Luckily, I've learned that I can reap many of the same benefits from *mini*-meditations and mindfulness practices as others do from lengthy meditation sessions. You, too, may find that mini-meditations fit smoothly into your daily life.

Mini-meditations, just like their longer cousins, *do* involve learning how to be mindful. Mindfulness pioneer Jon Kabat-Zinn defines mindfulness as "paying attention on purpose, in the present moment, and non-judgmentally." In addition, mindfulness "is an open, compassionate attitude toward your inner experience," as *Psychology Today* blogger Melanie Greenberg writes in *The Stress-Proof Brain*.

No matter how busy you are, you have time for the mini-meditations below—each takes 30 seconds or less.

12 Mindful Mini-Meditations

1. **Recognize the signs of your personal stress response.** Is your mind racing? Is your heart rate elevated? Are your fists clenched? Train yourself to use

stress as a cue that you need to put one or more of the actions below into effect. Just noticing your stress can help you feel better, once you realize that you have a choice of what to do about it.

2. **Take one or more deep breaths.** You just tried this, and it worked—and it works wherever you are, whether in your cubicle at work, at a family dinner, in your car, or waiting in line. Even one deep breath lets your body know that you are turning off the "fight-or-flight" response and turning on the "rest-and-restore" system. Deep, relaxing breaths also take the edge off anxiety, slowing the heart rate and lowering blood pressure. The decision to take a few deep breaths is a powerful way to help yourself get back in control. All the mini-meditations below will be more effective with deliberate breathing.

3. **Put your emotions into words.** "Stressed." "Anxious." "Furious." *Labeling* your emotions has an immediate calming effect. Why? Putting words to feelings shifts some of your brain activity from the emotional areas to the thinking areas of your brain. Then you can problem-solve.

4. **Open your eyes.** During your mini-meditation, you can keep your eyes open. I had no idea that eyes-open meditation was even possible, let alone desirable. But Pema Chodron, in her book *How to Meditate*, gives instructions for mindfulness meditation that includes this tip:

> Open the eyes, because it furthers this idea of wakefulness. We are not meditating in hopes of going further into sleep, so to speak...This isn't a transcendental type of meditation where you're trying to go into special states of consciousness. Rather, we meditate to become completely open to life. So keeping the eyes

open actually demonstrates this intention to stay with the present. It is a gesture of openness.

You may find that opening your eyes helps you open your mind. One further advantage: No one needs to know that you are secretly meditating. Of course, meditating with eyes closed is also a possibility. Experiment and see what works best for you.

5. **Choose one activity to do with mindful attention.** You can do any activity mindfully: Walking in nature, talking with a spouse or child, taking a shower, even sitting in a meeting—these activities can be done with deliberate intent to focus on the present moment. The classic exercise is to focus on your breathing; when you focus on the breath, you take a momentary break from worrying about the future or obsessing about the past.

6. **Offer yourself some mindful self-compassion.** If you notice that your mind is conjuring up scenarios that make you anxious or angry, give yourself some reassuring words. A little self-compassion goes a long way to calm an agitated spirit. "May I be kind to myself in this difficult moment" is an example of compassionate self-talk that is short and soothing.

7. **Accept your thoughts as "just thoughts."** As you go through your day, you may notice that your mind often creates disturbing mental stories and scenarios. That's because, to quote Zen practitioner Jack Kornfield, "The mind has no shame." When these odd or upsetting thoughts come up, neutralize them by telling yourself, *"Just thoughts."* Then take a deep breath to counter any stress that your mental chatter may have caused and re-focus on the present moment.

8. **Practice watching your thoughts pass by, as if you were watching a parade.** By witnessing your thoughts and emotions, you can discover a lot about

urself—your preoccupations, needs, worries, and
dues, among others. Some themes will emerge over
and over. You will also begin to notice that your
emotions and thoughts change and dissolve over
time. "This too shall pass" is a motto that accurately
describes the flow of our mental activity. You don't
have to join the parade of thoughts; you can just
watch it go by. Take what Greenberg calls "an observ-
ing stance."

9. **Smile a little bit.** If you've ever noticed statues of the
meditating Buddha, you may wonder why there is a
half-smile on his face. Why is the Buddha smiling?
A smile can magically relax your mind and body. Try
it. You can feel your facial muscles respond with an
immediate release of tension.

10. **Practice the "Notice 5 Things" exercise.** If you want
to tune in to your surroundings, decide to notice five
interesting things you can see, hear, feel, or smell. This
simple exercise will enliven any routine activity, such
as a walk, by inviting you to notice what is unique,
new, or previously unseen. It's literally an eye-opener.

11. **Recite a calming motto, mantra, or prayer.** Write
down a few perspective-giving sayings, tape them up,
and read them to yourself when needed. "The Serenity
Prayer" works for many people. You might also think
of something a parent, friend, or colleague told you
that brought you calm and reassurance.

12. **Focus on gratitude.** Stop your stress by taking 30
seconds to focus on a few things for which you are
grateful. Noticing the positive things in your life,
paired with a few deep breaths, is the perfect recipe
for a calmer mind and body.

What works for you?

Some of these 12 mini-meditations require practice and persistence. But the rewards are great—less stress, more awareness of the present moment, and less self-caused mental suffering. So if you can't, or don't want to, carve out time for formal meditation, try one of the mini-meditations above or create your own. Experiment and figure out what helps you.

© Meg Selig. Posted Mar 01, 2017 on psychologytoday.com.

References

Chodron, Pema (2013). *How to Meditate,* Boulder: Sounds True.

Greenberg, Melanie (2016). *The Stress-Proof Brain,* Oakland, CA: New Harbinger.

"The mind has no shame." Quoted in Bernhard, T. (2010). How to Be Sick, Somerville, MA: Wisdom Publications.

Vacation. Tello, M. "Regular meditation more beneficial than vacation." Harvard Health Letter, Oct. 27, 2016.

CHAPTER 15

"MOVEMENT IS MEDICINE:" A MOTTO WORTH MEMORIZING

Do you have arthritis, Parkinson's disease, type 2 diabetes, depression, or other health conditions? Here's what can help.

"Movement is medicine."

This motto summarizes in three words a conclusion of numerous research studies. Movement—everything from fidgeting to low-impact aerobics to high-intensity interval training—can prevent some diseases, ease the symptoms of others, and even reverse some chronic conditions.

"Movement is Medicine": The Evidence

Here are just a few headlines from hundreds of recent studies that spotlight the role of movement in curing or easing the symptoms of various diseases and conditions. (While most studies do not prove that movement causes these positive changes, all show that exercising and activity are highly correlated with them.)

1. Physical activity can improve arthritis symptoms by 40%.

2. Exercise alleviates some symptoms of Parkinson's disease and can slow its progression. As health writer Jane Brody explains, regular exercise, tailored to the needs of Parkinson's patients, "can result in better posture; less stiffness; improved flexibility of muscles and joints; faster and safer walking ability; less difficulty performing the tasks of daily living; and an overall higher quality of life."

3. Exercise can reduce your risk of developing type 2 diabetes. Specifically, following the public health recommendation to exercise moderately for 150 minutes a week can cut your risk of developing type 2 diabetes by 26%, according to a recent study which summarized data from over a million people. Any amount of exercise, however, was helpful in reducing risk.

4. Sitting too much for too long increases the risk of dying early. Why? Sitting for prolonged periods reduces blood flow to the legs and increases the risk of heart disease by accelerating the build-up of plaque in the arteries. Constant sitting also puts people at higher risk for diabetes, depression, and obesity.

   You may have to stay seated for most of your eight-hour workday. But all is not lost. As reported in the *Harvard Health Blog*, as little as 25 minutes of moderate activity a day can offset some of the negative effects of eight hours of sitting. Moreover, 60-75 minutes of activity per day eliminates the risk of death entirely, even in those who sit for more than eight hours or more.

5. Older women who sit too much and exercise too little show biological aging at the cellular level. Cells of sedentary women have shorter telomeres, tiny caps at the end of DNA strands that protect chromosomes from deterioration and premature aging.

6. Standing up and walking around for five minutes every hour improves health and well-being. A study of desk workers concluded: "Standing up and walking around for five minutes every hour during the work-day could lift your mood, combat lethargy without reducing focus and attention, and even dull hunger pangs, according to an instructive new study."

7. Both aerobic exercise and weight training appear to cause striking improvements in brain health and thinking skills; they also can slow age-related decline in memory.

8. Twenty minutes of exercise can act as an anti-inflammatory. It's encouraging that even a 20-minute walk can produce anti-inflammatory effects by stimulating the immune system.

9. Exercise can boost your mental health. Exercise can counter depression, stress, and anxiety, according to an increasing body of research. The Anxiety and Depression Association of America reports that regular exercise can work as well as medication for some people who suffer from anxiety and depression. (Note: Do not stop taking medication without consulting with your doctor.)

10. Physical activity was associated with a lower risk of 13 types of cancer. This conclusion was from a large-scale study that analyzed data from over a million people.

Various other benefits of exercise and physical activity have been well documented over the years. Exercise may strengthen bones and preserve muscle mass, thereby lowering your risk for falls and fractures. Exercise can help you lose weight or maintain a healthy weight, indirectly reducing your risk of type 2 diabetes. Exercise can prevent or ameliorate back pain, as I well know from personal experience. Moderate exercise can rev up the immune system, helping us fight off colds. Studies suggest that exercise lifts mood, raises feelings of satisfaction and self-esteem, and even makes you happier.

Most of the above benefits do not demand Herculean exercise efforts. In most cases, even small increments of activity were shown to have a positive effect. Small steps toward a more active life transform into big health gains over time.

> "When we get stiff, achy and sluggish, we generally don't recognize these signals as cues that our body craves movement. Instead, we misinterpret them as a need for rest, which makes us stiffer, achier and even more sluggish."
> —Carol and Mitchell Krucoff, authors of *Healing Moves*

Mini-Goals

You don't need to become an obsessive exerciser to use movement as your medicine. Try these mini-goals:

1. Find a motivator. Is it long life, more energy, less pain, or something else? Feel free to adopt "Movement is medicine" as your personal motto to motivate yourself to persist. Or maybe you like this one: "Motion is lotion."

2. Begin interpreting stiffness, aches and pains, and lethargy as cues to move around, **not** as signals to sit and rest. This helpful idea comes from Carol and Mitchell Krucoff, authors of *Healing Moves*.

3. Get up every hour and walk around or stretch for five minutes.

4. Mark off times on your calendar for your "appointments" with exercise.

5. If you are not an exerciser yet, begin with small doses of exercise, say, 5-15 minutes a day of walking or your favorite moderate aerobic activity. Gradually build up to 150 minutes a week (the standard public health recommendation). Or just do a little better than before.

6. Enjoy "exercise snacks," small bites of movement that keep your blood moving. Stretch, walk around the room, stand up, or find an excuse to walk up the stairs.

Cautions

Since exercise is medicine, remember to take the proper dose. Most people "under-dose" on exercise, but you can also overdose on it, just as you can OD on any medication. With the help of your doctor, decide what kind of movement might be medicine for you. Of course, exercise is not a cure-all. Those who have certain diseases or chronic conditions might not benefit from exercise at all, be unable to do it at all, or experience harms from it.

I also would not want to contribute to "the blame game." There are so many factors at play when it comes to illnesses and disease that it would be off-base to shine a spotlight of blame on someone's exercise and health practices. Genetics is a powerful player, even at times determining whether you respond well to exercise or are a "non-responder."

Exercise is of vital importance but must be balanced with other meaningful activities such as friendship, family, work, and pleasure. Taking breaks, rest, and good sleep are essential to health and happiness, also.

Movement Can Be More Than Medicine

Exercising can be a pleasurable experience when you discover the motions that your body enjoys. May you find exercise that brings you health, happiness, and the pure joy of moving with ease!

© Meg Selig. Posted on psychologytoday.com, March 30, 2017.

References

Krucoff, Carol and Mitchell, "9 Steps to Harness the Power of Physical Activity," healingwell.com, 8.22.2018.

Nakvi, Jia. "Arthritis afflicts 1 in 4 adults in the U.S., CDC report finds." *Washington Post*, 3.7.2017.

Brody, J. "Exercise Can Be a Boon to People with Parkinson's Disease." *New York Times*, 1.23.2017.

"Some is good. More is better. Regular exercise can cut your diabetes risk." *ScienceDaily*, 10.18.2016.

Bakalar, N. "Sitting Increases the Risk of Dying Early." *New York Times*, 3.29.2016.

Telomeres. "Too much sitting, too little exercise may accelerate biological aging." *ScienceDaily*, 1.18.2017.

"Exercise ... It does a body good: 20 minutes can act as anti-inflammatory." *ScienceDaily*, 1.12.2017.

"Physical activity associated with lower risk of many cancers." *ScienceDaily*, 5.16.2016.

CHAPTER 16

TALKING BACK TO CHRONIC PAIN

Can you reduce chronic pain by changing your self-talk? If you are over 65 and reading this essay, it is likely that you have some sort of chronic pain. Chronic pain is a widespread problem, afflicting between 60 and 75% of older adults in the U.S. A well-established technique for managing this pain is daily physical activity.

However, a recent (2020) study in the journal *Pain* described a vicious cycle in which some pain sufferers refrained from physical activity because of pain, thereby increasing their pain problems, raising their risk of depression, and worsening their general health because of adopting a more sedentary lifestyle. As movement experts Mitchell and Carol Krucoff say, "When we get stiff, achy and sluggish, we generally don't recognize these signals as cues that our body craves movement. Instead, we misinterpret them as a need for rest, which makes us stiffer, achier and even more sluggish."

143 pain sufferers (all of whom had knee osteoarthritis) were recruited for the study. They all wore accelerometers which measured their activity levels and wrote in their journals each morning about how much pain they were experiencing. Some participants wrote comments that sounded desperate like:

- "The pain is terrible and is not going to get any better."
- "I can't stand the pain anymore."

The researchers labeled this kind of talk "catastrophizing," defined as feeling an extreme sense of hopelessness or help-lessness. Such catastrophizing self-talk was independent of participants' actual experience of pain.

The researchers suggested that further research might be able to help chronic pain sufferers view their pain differently by altering their self-talk, but did not explain how they would do this.

I think I can help them out, with the assistance of chronic pain expert Toni Bernhard. Bernhard is the author of *How to Be Sick* and numerous other books about chronic illness. She warns that chronic pain sufferers and those who care about them must be careful not to buy into the unrealistic belief that "perfect health is within your power if you'd just eat right, exercise, etc." This view is not only simplistic but is actively harmful because it holds pain sufferers to unrealistic standards.

That said, there are indeed more skillful ways to practice better self-talk. Here are a few tips from Bernhard:

1. Eliminate emotionally charged adjectives like "terrible" and "unbearable." These loaded terms can increase the mental suffering you may feel. Instead, describe your symptoms in a neutral way: "Pain is here today."

2. Remind yourself that pain levels fluctuate throughout the day, and even change minute by minute.

3. Use self-talk that gently challenges your hopeless and helpless feelings:

- "It's not true that the pain will never get better. There are good times and bad times."
- "Even a little exercise might increase my mobility."
- "Avoiding physical activity may feel good in the short run but isn't good for me in the long run."
- "I can't control the pain, but I can control my response to it."
- Create a mantra that would work for you. My mantra: "Any amount of exercise is better than no exercise at all."

In addition to self-talk solutions, you might try behavior solutions. For easy and fun examples of these, take a look at the next chapter on "Exercise Snacks."

Since the research above applied only to people with osteoarthritis, it might not apply to your particular health condition. All the more reason to heed this warning: If you are chronically ill, don't engage in self-blame. And if you are not chronically ill, don't judge others who are. There are lots of moving parts to this situation.

© Meg Selig, 2020.

References

Bergland, C. "The Domino Effect of Daily Pain Catastrophizing," psychologytoday.com, 8.26.2020.

Bernhard, T. (2020) *How to Be Sick: Your Pocket Companion.* Wisdom Publications: Somerville, MA.

"Pain 'catastrophizing' may lead to little exercise, more time sedentary," ScienceDaily, August 27, 2020: https://www.sciencedaily.com/releases/2020/08/200825160549.htm

CHAPTER 17

10 DELICIOUS "EXERCISE SNACKS" FOR FUN AND FITNESS

The idea of "exercise snacks" can break down mental barriers to being active.

Have you had any delicious "exercise snacks" lately?

The phrase "exercise snacks" refers to small, even tiny, morsels of physical activity, such as standing for a few minutes after sitting for a while. The activity does not need to be lengthy, tiring, or involve formal exercise. It can be vigorous only if you choose to make it so.

I found the evocative phrase "exercise snacks" in a recent research report in ScienceDaily.com. The article described a 2019 study which linked three short bouts, or should I say "bites," of stair-climbing throughout the day with improved cardiovascular health. The stair-climbing took only about 20 seconds, yet after just six weeks participants increased their aerobic fitness by 5%, had stronger legs, and generated more power when cycling. That's a lot of benefits from just three tiny exercise snacks per day!

A smorgasbord of research studies suggests the same thing as the stair-climbing study above—that even small amounts of exercise can have a variety of positive health effects. A few examples from recent research:

- Just 10 minutes of slow cycling on a stationary bicycle improved memory and increased coordination in different parts of the brain in college students.
- Using a database of about 500,000 people from various studies, a review in *The Journal of Happiness Studies* discovered that just 10 minutes of exercise per day was enough to lift the mood of participants.
- Another study found that even five-minute bouts of exercise increased longevity and reduced the risk of premature death.
- Five minutes of moving around every hour can combat "sitting diseases" such as diabetes, atherosclerosis, and obesity and improve mood and alertness.

For certain health conditions, small portions of exercise are even better than one large "meal." For example, in a 2014 study, three short rounds of treadmill exercise before breakfast, lunch, and dinner were more effective in lowering blood sugar throughout the day than one 30-minute exercise session before dinner. In addition, a 2012 study found that three 10-minute morsels of exercise lowered blood pressure in participants more than one 30-minute session did.

Change Your Mindset, Improve Your Health

The phrase "exercise snacking" reminds us that we can view exercise as a treat. I love the phrase "exercise snack" because it is a powerful way to reframe our collective mindset about exercise. Too often people view exercise as a dreaded chore. The phrase "exercise snacking" reminds us that we can view exercise as a treat. Moving around can feel good and give us pleasure! And, by the way, if you think of a task as "fun," you will need less willpower to accomplish it.

The idea of exercise snacking also challenges the "all-or-nothing" mentality of "If I can't do my full workout today, I may as well do nothing." Rather, if you can develop the mindset of exercise snacking, you can tell yourself, "OK, I can't do my full workout, but I can treat myself to a few exercise snacks throughout the day."

Below are ideas for possible exercise snacks. While many of the exercise snacks in the research studies above were high intensity, the suggestions below focus on easy, low-intensity, mini-exercises. Still, you will reap amazing benefits over time. The key: Indulge in exercise snacks as frequently as possible and keep it going on a daily basis.

10 Yummy Exercises Snacks for Fun and Fitness

Try these tasty exercise snacks:

1. *Climb the stairs.* This is the classic exercise snack. Forgot something on the second floor? Fantastic! You get to run up and get it. If you can do it vigorously, so much the better, but you'll get a health benefit at any speed. I love stair-climbing, and I've found I can even use it as a cue to feel grateful for my good health.

2. *Fidget.* Tap your feet to the music, stretch a little, wiggle in your chair, change positions, do a little chair dance. All these mini-movements improve blood flow and alertness. Sitting still for long periods of time, whether at home or on an airplane, raises your risk for blood clots and other serious circulation problems.

3. *Get out of your chair and stand up. Then do it again.* Baseball great Satchel Paige once said: "I don't generally like running. I believe in training by rising gently up and down from the bench." The *Harvard Health*

Letter backs up Paige's idea. They recommend that you get up twice—get up, sit down, get up again. You'll strengthen your legs, abs, and hip muscles. If you try it, you'll see that this is an invigorating 5-second workout.

4. *Rub lotion into your skin.* Like me, you may view this chore as tedious, but if you look at it as an exercise snack, it becomes more worthwhile. Your skin and your body will thank you.

5. *Fetch the newspaper every morning.* I look forward to this task every day—I get to experience the weather, survey the neighborhood, savor the morning quiet, and get rid of a few aches and pains. (Of course to snack on this exercise, you must subscribe to a newspaper. Consider it a donation to support freedom of the press.)

6. *Walk in place while you watch TV.* During a commercial break, stand up. Or, even better, stand up and walk in place. You could set a standard for yourself: "Every half hour, I will stand up for one minute of commercials."

7. *Clean out a few items from your refrigerator or pantry.* That's right—do some exercise snacking to control food snacking. The irony is delicious! (If this activity would give you the munchies, skip it and try some of the other suggestions.)

8. *Stroll through your living quarters.* Meander around your house or apartment. Walk slowly from room to room—or just walk around the room. Pick up a piece of trash and toss it. Admire the photo of your family on the wall. Think of a décor improvement. Move a dish into the sink. Sit back down.

9. *Pay a bill, stand up, recycle.* Paying bills, making phone calls, hunting for a piece of information about trash pick-up on your city's website...writer Elizabeth Emens calls these tasks "Life Admin." I dislike these tasks so much that not having to do them anymore is on my list of "Three Good Things About Death." But since you have no choice about Life Admin, make it fun. After paying a bill, stand up and stroll over to your recycling box—which you have strategically placed across the room.

10. *Do any household chore.* Light house-keeping helps you burn a few calories while getting things done. Bonus: Research shows that doing the dishes mindfully will lower stress.

Of course, there are an infinite number of possible exercise snacks. The above list is just meant to jog your brain (pun intended) for ideas that would work best for you.

Small Wins

No amount of exercise, however small, is ever wasted.

Sometimes you need an exercise meal instead of an exercise snack. It's true that you can get more fitness benefits with consistent moderate to vigorous exercise. For maximum benefit, the World Health Organization recommends 150 minutes of exercise per week (say, 30 minutes/day, 5 days/week).

But exercise snacks are beneficial, too. Not only do they improve mood, fitness, and overall health, like all "small wins," they can have a ripple effect, motivating you to keep moving and improving. Small daily improvements in your well-being may encourage you to exercise more, even to create the exercise habit. As author James Clear points out in his book *Atomic Habits*, we too often underestimate the power of making small improvements on a daily basis. Further, he argues that "The seed of every habit is a single, tiny decision."

Can you make a "single, tiny decision" to indulge in a few more exercise snacks each day?

© Meg Selig. Posted on psychologytoday.com, Jan 29, 2019.

References

Clear, J. (2018). *Atomic Habits*. NY: Penguin Random House.

Combat "sitting diseases." Reynolds, G. "Work. Walk 5 minutes. Work." *New York Times*, Dec. 28, 2016.

Stairclimbing. https://www.sciencedaily.com/ releases/2019/01/190118110833.htm, 2019.

Stand up. "5 minute fixes for better health," *The Harvard Health Letter*, Dec. 2018.

CHAPTER 18

MY TWO FRONT TEETH: A PERSONAL ESSAY ON VANITY

I've always been self-conscious about my huge two front teeth. When I was growing up, we called them "buck teeth," an apt label for teeth that seemed to kick right out of your mouth. Even after some orthodontia in junior high school, never fully completed, my front teeth seemed to dominate my face when I smiled.

It took me until I became a senior to re-visit this issue. No, not a senior in high school or college, a senior over the age of 65. I had discovered that the aging of my face was a source of distress and was casting about for simple solutions. My goal was to improve my appearance without a facelift, having learned that a so-called "mini-facelift" was major surgery—a four-five hour procedure requiring intubation and anesthesia. Vain as I am, I didn't entirely rule out a facelift, but I thought I would try other, less drastic, procedures.

I began to notice and inwardly wail over those prominent front teeth once again. I timidly asked my dentist if it were possible to file down the offending teeth.

"Of course!" he exclaimed. "And I think you would look and feel much better with this simple procedure. In fact, we could even file off your front lower teeth as well."

Even better! My lower teeth were smaller but uneven and jagged. If those teeth could be corrected, too, I would be ecstatic.

I learned from my dentist and from a little Internet research that:

- "Teeth contouring" is a common procedure.
- There is little risk involved.
- It can be performed without anesthesia.
- Price: $450 at my dentist's office.

On the day of my appointment, I took a "before" photo of myself and my humongous teeth. What would they look like "after?"

At my appointment, my dentist and I agreed on a "less is more" approach. He would file down the two front teeth so that they were more approximate in size to the two teeth on either side of them but would stop after each filing so I could look and assess.

Each filing took about 30 seconds. After each, I glanced critically at my teeth. Better and better! Little by little, the dentist gradually reduced the size of my incisors and, as much as humanly possible, corrected the snaggle-toothed appearance of my lower front four teeth.

At the end of our appointment, I was beside myself with joy. "I am so happy!" I told my dentist. "Thank you so much!" As I walked out, his very efficient office staff unloaded $450 from my credit card.

Back home again, I compared my mouth with the photo I had taken. There was little difference. My front teeth snugly topped my lower lip when I smiled, as usual. There was considerable improvement in the lowers, with a more even, though far from perfect, appearance. But how often do you notice someone's lower teeth?

Over the weeks that followed, not one person ever commented that my smile looked different in any way. Yet I felt different and better. In fact, I felt a remarkable increase in self-confidence, especially considering the modest nature of this procedure.

A skeptical part of me wondered, "Have I been bewitched? Was this all done with smoke and mirrors? Did I just pay $450 to feel better without really looking better?" It's humbling to think that I, like the emperor in the Hans Christian Anderson story, might have been the victim of a swindle, aided and abetted by my own vanity. At one point I even wondered if the dentist had filed down the teeth at all or had simply turned on his whirring machine and pretended to do it.

It didn't matter. The feeling of self-confidence remained, and it was priceless. Who cares if anyone noticed but me? Months later, I'm still happy I had the procedure. I may look almost the same, but, magic or not, I feel like a million bucks.

One Small Spark:

A Peculiar Question

With a head so congested that I couldn't hear properly, I decided I'd better get help at a walk-in clinic one weekend day. It was during the COVID crisis, so I was wearing a mask.

The nurse ushered me into a room. A few minutes later she returned to ask me the usual medical questions. Except that this question was one I hadn't heard in a very long time: "So, Mrs. Selig, what was the date of your last menstrual period?"

I paused, milking the situation for all it was worth. "Hmm," I said. "Let me think. Oh, it was approximately 25 years ago. And you have just made my day." We enjoyed a good laugh together.

There are lots of advantages to wearing a mask.

CHAPTER 19

THE ESSENTIAL MENTAL HABIT FOR HEALTH AND HAPPINESS AT ANY AGE

"Enjoy the little things, for one day you may look back and realize they were the big things."
— Robert Brault

The Power of a Keystone Habit

What if you decided to change one simple habit and discovered that your life became better in all sorts of ways that you never could have predicted?

Such is the case when you adopt a "keystone habit." Keystone habits are those that spark a cascade of positive changes, often unrelated to the original change. These chain reactions "help other good habits take hold," writes Charles Duhigg in *The Power of Habit*.

There is a *mental* keystone habit that is highly related to longevity, happiness, and health among older people. That habit is **gratitude.** At any age, cultivating the attitude of gratitude can trigger both other helpful mental habits and seemingly unrelated behavior habits. Below I'll reveal the direct benefits of practicing gratitude as well as the unexpected and sometimes incredible "keystone benefits."

Gratitude Over Despair

Catastrophic fantasies. Angry scenarios replayed again and again. Repetitive negative thoughts. There are swarms of negative thinking habits that waste time, cause stress and suffering, and sap you of self-esteem and self-compassion. Since it's hard to change those slippery old patterns, simply replace some of them with a positive thinking pattern instead—like the keystone habit of gratitude.

Training yourself to focus on gratitude is relatively easy. One method is to keep a gratitude journal, noting on a regular basis what you are thankful for. Another method is to practice the iconic "Three Good Things" exercise. In this exercise, every night for one week, you either write down or mentally note three good things that happened that day, along with your best guess as to why they happened. I find that a once-a-week refresher keeps my head on straight. Or just develop the habit of "counting your blessings" as they occur.

You can also use a cue to remind yourself to feel grateful. When I bound up the stairs to fetch something I've forgotten, I feel grateful that my chronic plantar fasciitis has abated for the time being, and that I can still climb stairs with ease at my age. While my health is not as good as it used to be, I can use "stair-climbing" as a reminder to appreciate the physical strengths I still have.

Direct benefits. It's not surprising that "the gratitude attitude" affects other mental habits. When your mind is filled with gratitude, there's less psychic space for negative thoughts and feelings. The conscious and deliberate practice of gratitude also triggers the following beneficial changes, according to psychologist Robert A. Emmons, author of *Thanks! How Practicing Gratitude Can Make You Happier*:

- Gratitude boosts happiness levels. In fact, cultivating the gratitude attitude actually raises your happiness set-point, according to Emmons. And happiness can increase life expectancy by as much as nine years, according to some estimates.
- Gratitude increases other positive emotions, such as joy, optimism, pleasure, and enthusiasm.
- Gratitude reduces depression and blocks negative emotions like envy and resentment.
- Gratitude leads people to become more optimistic about the future.

Keystone benefits. Gratitude practice also has an amazing "spark" effect. For example, research indicates that:

- People who keep gratitude journals on a regular basis exercise more regularly. Now *that* is synergy!
- People who keep gratitude journals report fewer health problems and recover more quickly from illness.
- Gratitude can strengthen self-control, according to the work of psychologist David DeSteno.
- Gratitude also increases patience, thereby reducing impulse buying and increasing saving behaviors.
- Gratitude strengthens relationships, by helping us acknowledge when others have helped us.
- Gratitude helps people rebound from stressful, even traumatic, situations.

The Gratitude Attitude

Keystone habits can vary from person to person. You might clean out one junk drawer and find yourself keeping better financial records and losing weight. Walking for twenty minutes a day could lift your mood and inspire you to create a mural for a community center. A keystone habit that transformed my life was quitting smoking. I became fascinated with how to change a habit and eventually taught a class, created a curriculum book, and wrote a book—all on the subject of successful habit change.

So, if you desire a thinking habit that will keep you happier, healthier, and give you more perspective on your life and relationships, make the choice to practice gratitude.

© Meg Selig. First published on psychologytoday.com, Jan 23, 2015. Revised 2020.

References

Keystone habits. Duhigg, C. (2012). *The Power of Habit.* (NY: Random House), pp.109 ff.

Three good things. Selig, M. (2010). *Changepower! 37 Secrets to Habit Change Success.* (NY: Taylor & Francis). p. 221, 246.

DeSteno, D. "How to Defeat the Impulse Buy." *New York Times,* Nov. 21, 2014.

Gratitude journals, etc. Emmons, Robert A. (2007). *Thanks! How the New Science of Gratitude Can Make You Happier.* (NY: Houghton Mifflin), p. 11 ff.

CHAPTER 20

THE HIDDEN COSTS OF NOISE POLLUTION

These 10 simple habits can protect your hearing.

The Surprising Harms of Our "Noise Habits"

My body was vibrating. My ears were ringing. My brain was numb. My heart was pounding.

No, I was not ill, nor had I just fallen in love. I was still experiencing the after-effects of a one-hour dinner in a high-noise environment—a sports bar with loud raucous talk and laughter augmented by chukka-chukka music in the background that our waiter insisted could not be turned down. I was surprised—and angry—at how painful just one hour of noise pollution could be.

This experience motivated me to question our "noise habits." What were the side effects of exposure to such ear-splitting cacophony? And what can we do to protect our hearing?

The U.S. Environmental Protection Agency (EPA) defines "noise" as "unwanted or disturbing sound." Since we can't see noise, we are often oblivious to its effects on us, even if the noise is "wanted." But the major side-effects of noise pollution are serious and sometimes surprising. The three most shocking facts I discovered are:

1. The top *preventable* cause of hearing loss is **noise**.

2. Excessive noise can lead to a whole host of other serious health problems. These include coronary artery disease, high blood pressure, stress-related health conditions such as migraine, colitis, and ulcers, and decreased sleep and sleep quality.

3. Excessive noise can lead to emotional problems such as mental fatigue, anxiety, and aggression.

How does noise pollution cause hearing loss? According to the National Institute on Deafness and Other Communication Disorders (NIDCD), sounds that are too loud or last for too long damage the hair cells in our ears that are responsible for transmitting sound to the brain. These hair cells are sensitive and, once damaged, cannot grow back.

Why is excessive noise hazardous to your physical health? The reason is that noise causes a stress response. You hear a loud sound, and a stress cascade begins—adrenaline is released, blood vessels constrict, muscles tense, and blood pressure rises. We are not fully in control of this stress response: "Even though noise may have no relationship to danger, the body will respond automatically to noise as a warning signal."

Why is excessive noise hazardous to your emotional health? Noise is associated with increased aggression, decreased helpful behavior, reduced motivation and task performance, and even impaired cognitive development in children. Moreover, hearing loss, whether caused by noise pollution or aging, can be a psychological problem as well as a physical problem. A person who suffers from hearing loss may tend to isolate himself, feel lonely, and, in extreme cases, succumb more easily to depression. Recent research also links hearing loss to a higher risk for dementia.

How to Reduce Your Risk of Hearing Loss

Some age-related hearing loss is inevitable, but noise-induced hearing loss (NIHL) is 100% preventable. Once it occurs, you can't reverse it, but you can prevent your hearing from deteriorating further. Here are ten habits that will reduce your risk:

1. Do a simple noise assessment in your home or office from time to time throughout the day. Stop for a moment. Listen. Is there background noise that could be eliminated or ameliorated? (Did you leave the sprinkler on?!)

2. Avoid places with a high noise level or limit your exposure.

3. When you find yourself raising your voice over noise, that's a clue that noise pollution could be harming your hearing. Beat a hasty retreat if you can.

4. Wear ear plugs (which fit in the ear) or headphones (which fit over the ear) in sound-polluted environments. Plan to bring noise-cancelling plugs/headphones when noise is unavoidable, such as on airplane flights.

5. Plan for "quiet time" every day. Give yourself a break, even from "good noise" (sorry about the oxymoron) such as your beloved music. Turn off the TV for a while.

6. Avoid ear-busters such as hair dryers, food processors, and leaf-blowers, or use them sparingly or with ear protection. This is not a trivial suggestion. The level at which noise can cause permanent hearing loss begins at about 85 decibels, typical of a hair dryer, food processor or kitchen blender.

7. Buy appliances with low noise ratings. If you have a timer on your dishwasher, set it so you will be away from the kitchen while it does its dirty work.

8. Turn down the volume on TVs, portable music players, and other sound systems. How low can you go and still hear comfortably? Experiment.

9. Protect children. Noisy environments affect children's ability to learn and their ability to cope with normal challenges. Educate children about caring for their ears.

10. Walk away from noise: If the outside environment is noisy, go inside and/or close windows. If the inside environment is noisy, go out.

The damage from most temporary noise exposure is reversible. So, driving down the highway singing loudly to your favorite music is not likely to hurt you. But when does too much noise lead to *irreversible* damage? If you are curious about the level of noise that can cause hearing damage, find the CDC's "noise meter" at their website. This clever meter illustrates how intensity and duration of sound combine to produce risk of hearing loss. You'll learn, among other things, that using a chain saw for more than two minutes without hearing protection is dangerous to your ears.

As for me, I survived the din of dinner. After just one hour of exposure, I was at little risk for permanent hearing loss. My server may not be so lucky. Unremitting noise exposure, day after day, provokes changes that are deafening, literally and figuratively. In fact, at least one study found that one third of students who work in noisy environments like music clubs, bars, and restaurants were found to have permanent hearing loss. Hearing loss is also an occupational hazard for construction workers, landscapers, and anyone who uses noisy machinery. (To file a complaint about hazardous noise in the workplace, contact OSHA.) Astonishingly, 1/5 of Americans over the age of 12 suffer from some hearing loss.

And as for the noisy restaurant—I'm going to follow my own advice in habit #2 and avoid it like the plague in the future.

© Meg Selig. Posted Sep 25, 2013, on psychologytoday.com.

References

*The leading cause of hearing loss…*Brody, J. "What causes hearing loss?" New York Times, March 25, 2013.

Noise as a warning signal. Chepesiuk, R. (2005). "Decibel Hell: The Effects of Living in a Noisy World." *https://www.ncbi.nlm.nih.gov/pmc/articles/PMC1253729/*

Goines, L. & Hagler, L. (2007). "Noise Pollution: A Modern Plague." *https://www.nonoise.org/library/smj/smj.htm*

CHAPTER 21

"WHAT?!:" LIFE WITH A HARD-OF-HEARING MAN

Recently, I was whispering a sweet nothing to my partner Brian. He responded, "WHAT?! What did you say?"

I answered loudly, "I SAID, I STILL FIND YOU ADORABLE AFTER ALL THESE YEARS."

Somehow a sweet nothing loses quite a lot of its original meaning when it is yelled. In fact, I felt almost angry. I had raised my voice, and that's what humans do when they are angry. My tenderness turned quickly into irritation.

Coping with an extremely hard-of-hearing partner requires creative problem-solving. Among the many things I have learned, three guidelines stand out: 1. Don't take it personally. 2. Maintain a sense of humor. 3. Use logistics and technology.

Since Brian has tried hearing aids without experiencing improvement in his hearing, there's no real solution to the "sweet nothings" problem except for me to get in the habit of speaking more clearly and emphatically and, most of all, directly into his ear when possible. I worry about his future brain health, since hearing loss is associated with cognitive decline. Happily, we've figured out other ways to adapt.

When we go to restaurants, we try to get a table where we can sit side by side. This way I can speak directly into Brian's ear. If we are given a four-top, that's OK, too. We do not sit across from each other—which would require hollering if the noise level is at all above normal. Instead, we sit right by each other. Sitting close together not only facilitates communication; it also facilitates hand-holding and other affectionate forms of touching that can substitute for speech.

But sometimes we find ourselves at opposite ends of a longish two-top. If it's noisy, we may resort to losing ourselves separately in our cellphones, which is why I do not judge when I see others looking at their phones rather than at each other. Each of us can be reasonably content reading from, say, the *New York Times* app (me) or checking the latest sports scores (him). By the way, sports is one of the easiest topics to discuss in this situation. You might not want to discuss the most recent email from your son or daughter, since you would have to shout it from the treetops. But yelling out, "Did you read about the latest trade?" is fairly harmless.

Many couples in our situation quarrel about how high the sound on the TV should be. We are no exception. However, thanks to the feature that assigns a number to each degree of volume, we can usually compromise. For example, I might request, "Could you turn it down to 12?"

I have also accepted that often I will need to assume the "translator" role. My basic technique resembles the *Saturday Night Live* Garrett Morris School of Sign-Language Interpretation—i.e., make your hands into a megaphone and shout. In a typical situation, a server at a restaurant might say, "Hi, my name is Britney, and I'll be your server today. Can I start you off with a beverage?"

"What?!" exclaims Brian.

I shout, "WHAT WOULD YOU LIKE TO DRINK?"

I am well-trained for the translator role since my father also became extremely hard of hearing as he aged. I have even learned to watch Brian's face for signs of incomprehension. When I see them, I'll ask, "Did you get what he said?" He'll say no, and I'll raise the volume two ticks on my own voice to explain the conversation, the joke, or the juicy piece of information that I know he'll enjoy.

Being hard of hearing is hard to live with sometimes, but it's a lot easier than many other problems of aging, so I consider myself lucky. I SAID, I CONSIDER MYSELF LUCKY.

© Meg Selig, 2019.

CHAPTER 22

50 YEARS, SAME HEALTHY WEIGHT, MY SECRETS

A weight loss of 10-15 pounds may seem trivial. But even minor weight loss can lead to health benefits.

A Promise to Myself

"The freshman 15." This phrase has come to denote what the typical college student gains during their freshman year of college. Funny thing: I actually did gain 15 pounds my freshman year. Not so funny: I was still 15 pounds overweight in my mid-20s.

I had not only gained weight; I had gained a dress size, too. I had slowed down a step and felt unhappy with my appearance.

So in 1970 I made a vow to lose the extra weight and maintain that weight loss for a lifetime.

This decision to change propelled me into a 50-year pattern of (mostly) healthy eating. From age 25 to age 75, my height (5'6") and weight (125) have remained almost the same. With 50 years at the same weight, I feel I've earned the street cred to share my secrets.

Why Worry About Weight?

My weight loss of 10-15 pounds may seem trivial. But even minor weight loss can lead to health benefits for a person who is overweight. The Center for Disease Control tells us: "Even a modest weight loss of 5 to 10 percent of your total body weight is likely to produce health benefits, such as improvements in blood pressure, blood cholesterol, and blood sugars." On the other hand, being overweight or obese is linked to a higher risk of numerous health problems, including type-2 diabetes, heart disease, some types of cancer, and, yes, even COVID-19.

Of course, I didn't know this information in 1970. I only knew that I wanted to feel better and look better.

This blog will describe why I gained weight, what I did to shed it, and alternative paths to a healthy weight.

Why Do College Students Gain Weight?

Seventy percent (70%!) of college students gain 13-47 pounds in college, so I was not the only one. Why? Late-night snacking, high-calorie dorm meals, and lack of exercise all take their toll, according to a 2012 study. The study showed that the "Freshman 15" was not a myth and could have lifelong health consequences.

My Motivators and Plan

My weight-loss method could be summed up as four "Ms" and one "P:" motivators, mindfulness, monitoring, moderation, and pleasure.

The first step toward change is to know your motivators. Mine were health, longevity, and looking better. Shallow though it may be, vanity can be a powerful motivator, especially when you are seeking a romantic partner, as I was.

Now I needed a plan. Since I desired lifelong weight control, I knew I had to avoid those two Dreadful Ds: Diet and Deprivation. Although the research on diets wasn't clear at that point (Now we know: Diets don't work in the long run.), I knew myself and realized that any eating plan based on self-denial was bound to fail. So I set about to create my own moderate eating plan, with the help of a few sensible nutrition books, like *Let's Eat Right to Keep Fit*, by Adele Davis, and *Diet for a Small Planet*, by Frances Moore Lappe.

I decided that one pillar of my plan would be *pleasure*. I would make every meal as healthy and pleasurable as possible, not denying myself any foods, just limiting the quantity. Plus, I would allow myself one sweet treat every day.

Fifty years ago, the word "mindfulness" had not yet come into currency. Though I didn't have the words for it, my goal was, in fact, *mindful eating*. I wanted to eat with awareness, enjoying my food, not gobbling it down. I made a pact with myself to refrain from what's now called "automatic eating," mindlessly munching one potato chip after another while watching TV, for example.

Armed with these ideas, vague though they were, I sallied forth to lose my extra 15 pounds.

The First Five Pounds

The first five pounds were a cinch. A friend once told me, "I'd rather eat my calories than drink them." That was an "aha" moment. My simple and painless plan: stop drinking soda. I substituted water and sparkling water. And bingo! Five pounds gone within one month. (Other possibilities: Substitute fruit for high-calorie fruit juices. Limit alcoholic drinks.)

The Next Five Pounds

Losing the rest of the weight was much more of a challenge. I experimented with various helpful ideas. Here's a list of the most useful ones gleaned from 50 years of learning about food and health:

1. *Predictable eating times.* I never miss a meal, and I eat pretty much at the same time every day: breakfast at 7 am, lunch at noon, dinner at 6 pm, treat at 7 pm. Knowing when I will next eat helps me avoid the hunger panic that leads to snacking.

2. *Eat with comfort.* Sit down. Eat slowly. Savor your food. It's all about pleasure.

3. *Know your daily calorie goal.* Most women should aim for a 2000 calorie/day diet. That means about 600 calories per meal, plus a 200-calorie treat. (For men, it's 2500 calories.) Thanks to Obamacare, chain restaurants must now provide calorie counts, helping all of us target that 600-calorie meal.

4. *Learn about serving sizes.* I learned that a serving of nuts should be about ¼ cup, for example. My first reaction: "That small!?" But now it seems just right. (For easy ways to remember serving sizes, consult the Mayo Clinic website.) There's no need to count calories. Just read the nutrition label on a few favorite foods, and you'll get a sense of how many calories you are consuming each day.

5. *Avoid automatic eating.* Eat at the table, not in front of the TV. Don't eat standing up. Think "pleasure."

6. *Limit snacking.* I stopped buying snack foods such as potato chips and pretzels, allowing myself to eat them only on special occasions. I reminded myself that meals were more enjoyable when I was hungry for them. Or, as my mother used to say, "Don't spoil your appetite!" And speaking of special occasions...

7. *Make some foods "special occasion foods."* With the exception of soda, I didn't eliminate any foods from my diet. Certain fattening foods, like mashed potatoes, biscuits, and rolls, became "special occasion" foods only, however.

8. *Ask yourself, "Is it worth the calories?"* I asked myself this question constantly to curb my intake of any foods that were just so-so. I learned to stop eating anything that wasn't tasty and resigned my membership in the Clean Plate Club.

9. *Follow the 20-minute rule.* The rule: It takes 10-20 minutes for your stomach to tell your brain that it's full. Can't decide whether to have seconds on something? Just wait a few minutes and see how you feel.

10. *Follow the 80% rule.* The rule: Aim to be 80% full, not 100% full. I love this rule! It reminds me that I do not need to stuff myself to feel satisfied.

11. *Monitor yourself.* I weighed myself regularly, reducing my food intake when I became 2-5 pounds over my goal weight (which happened often). (Note: Some people may find that frequent weighing can trigger unhealthy eating patterns or even eating disorders. If you think you might fall into this category, try another method of self-monitoring like keeping a food journal.)

12. *Eat more fruits and veggies.* Mediterranean-style eating plans, which emphasize grains, fruits, and veggies, are beneficial for your health.

13. *Enjoy regular exercise.* Exercise offers a smorgasbord of benefits. I aim for the World Health Organization standard of 150 minutes of moderate exercise per week.

14. *Shrug off slips.* The ability to bounce back from short-term failures may be the most significant predictor of long-term weight-loss success, according to cognitive therapist Judith Beck.

As time went on, I became savvier about choosing "whole foods" that were organic, lacked preservatives, and were free of strange chemicals with unknown health consequences. I adopted food writer Michael Pollan's famous motto: "Eat food. Not too much. Mostly plants."

Other People, Other Plans

Many people who tell me they have an unhealthy relationship with food may not be able to benefit from a self-directed, moderate eating plan. The more addiction-like your habit, the more you may need structure and support. Helpful support groups for weight loss and healthy eating include Weight-Watchers (now WW), TOPS (Take off Pounds Sensibly), and Overeaters Anonymous. Many people have benefited from the support and guidance of a therapist, health coach, or hospital-based weight-loss group.

Remember that weight loss is not necessarily the path to personal fulfillment.

Remember that weight loss is not necessarily the path to personal fulfillment. I lost weight in part to find a romantic partner, but in retrospect I'm sure that being ten pounds heavier would not have derailed my marriage.

The Last Five Pounds

And what did I do to work off that last five pounds? Nothing. I decided to be satisfied with my weight of 125, stop my nitpicking, and enjoy life. My motto for this and other health changes: "Don't let the perfect be the enemy of the good."

© Meg Selig. Posted August, 2020.

References

Modest weight loss. https://www.cdc.gov/healthyweight/losing_weight/index.html

COVID-19 and overweight: https://www.cdc.gov/coronavirus/2019-ncov/need-extra-precautions/people-with-medical-conditions.html

2012 study. https://www.health.com/family/college-gain-weight

Selig, M. Weigh or no weigh. https://www.psychologytoday.com/us/blog/changepower/201010/the-scale-friend-or-foe-college-students

Selig, M. "Why Diets Don't Work and What Does." https://www.psychologytoday.com/us/blog/changepower/201010/why-diets-dont-work-and-what-does

Selig, M. "Heathy Eating, For All the Right Reasons." https://www.psychologytoday.com/us/blog/changepower/201011/healthy-eating-all-the-right-reasons

CHAPTER 23

IS YOUR HOME A SAFETY HAZARD? 6 DANGERS FOR OLDER ADULTS…AND EVERYONE ELSE

> "We have met the enemy and he is us."
> — Pogo (cartoonist Walt Kelly)

Home sweet home? Not always.

It's April, 2020. Everyone is worried, and with good reason, about COVID-19 and the people who might be carriers. But if you are worried about your safety and health, keep in mind that sometimes the enemy is not "out there" but right at home. In fact, sometimes "we have met the enemy and he is us," as the cartoon character Pogo used to say.

To be clear: From everything the experts are telling us, the stay-at-home orders are the most powerful way to staunch the spread of COVID-19. So stay at home! But because of the "halo effect," you might see your good ol' home as a non-threatening environment. What could be more comforting and safe than your very own living space?

Actually, safety expert Steve Casden says, "It might be best to assume that everything in your house is trying to kill you." That includes kitchen knives, a broken wine glass, scented candles, and much more. He makes this argument in a deadly funny article entitled, appropriately, "Do Not Stand on That Chair." Among other dangers, he points to these common actions that can lead to injuries or other disasters:

- Using a chair instead of a stepladder to fetch something from a high shelf or cabinet.
- Using a kitchen knife incorrectly or carelessly.
- Forgetting to turn off a burner on the stove.
- Neglecting to blow out a candle.

He also noted that the coronavirus crisis is an especially bad time to become a victim of your own carelessness: "Without a functioning health care system, an everyday injury could end your life. A pandemic is the time to start being a kind of careful that you've likely never considered before." You do not want to end up in the ER ever—but especially not right now when health care personnel may have other priorities. Moreover, you could get exposed to the very virus you are trying to avoid. (That said, do not avoid getting medical help for serious problems. Precautions are now in place to protect patients.)

6 Safety Challenges in Your Home

What "kind of careful" should you be during a crisis in which you are sheltering in place? For starters, avoid these six common ways to have an accident at home. (Note: I've focused on adults and older adults, but you might inspect your living space with an eye to child-proofing, too.)

1. Falling

Fall hazards can trip up children and adults of any age. However, older adults are particularly vulnerable to the life-threatening consequences of falls. For people over 50, falls are the leading cause of death from injuries. Almost 1 out of 10 people over the age of 50 will die within a month of surgery for a broken hip, according to an NPR report. One in 10!

To prevent falls, take these steps:

- Walk from room to room, noting any obstacles that could be trip hazards, especially those in high-traffic areas. Move or remove them.
- Hold onto the banister when going up or down stairs. Make sure it does not wiggle! If it does, get it fixed.
- Remove small area rugs. These are major slipping-and-tripping hazards.
- Light up dark areas of your home.
- Fix uneven stairs or steps. Install grab bars in critical areas of the home, such as showers.
- If you must stand on something to get an item from a high shelf, recruit another family member to stand by. At the very least, have your phone with you so you can call 911 in case of an accident.

2. Bump hazards

Coffee tables and other low tables, especially those with sharp corners, can be dangerous bump hazards for people of all ages. Install "corner guards" to protect babies, toddlers, and adults from head and limb injuries. Your open dishwasher door is also a sneaky bump hazard.

Bump hazards can lead to painful leg bruises or even deep gashes. If stitches are required, you'd need an ER visit—a bad idea right now.

And while we're looking at the dishwasher, remember to put the business end of your flatware face down. You want to grab the handles when you remove your knives and forks, not the blades or tines.

3. Eye hazards

Safety goggles or wraparound glasses can protect you when you are mowing the lawn, doing outdoor projects, using power tools, or tackling tough cleaning jobs. Wear glasses when handling any substances that pose eye dangers, such as polishes, ammonia, and bleach. (If you are out shopping, goggles or glasses might also afford some protection against virus droplets entering your eyes.)

4. Indoor air pollution

"If you are one of the millions of Americans breathing polluted air, you may be at a greater risk of catching the coronavirus and of having a more severe infection," according to a recent *New York Times* article. Why? For one, air pollution can aggravate chronic lung problems such as asthma and COPD. Also, exposure to air pollution raises the risk of damage to your immune and respiratory systems, making viral illnesses more toxic.

If pollution levels are high in your area, stay indoors. While outdoor air pollution may be out of your control, there are some ways to mitigate indoor pollution:

- When cleaning, painting, or using harmful chemicals, make sure you have good ventilation.
- Don't smoke in or near your house. In fact, don't smoke!
- When you cook, turn on the ventilation hood above your stove.
- Unless you live in a highly polluted area, open windows for fresh air.
- Buy an air purifier if you can afford it.
- Fix water damage to prevent mold.

5. Neglecting exercise and other healthy habits

Counterintuitive though it may seem, exercise reduces fall risks. That's because exercise promotes balance as well as strength and flexibility. So keep up your regular exercise program. But if that's impossible, just do what you can. Even small "exercise snacks" like getting up and moving around every hour, doing chores, and taking brief walks can lift your mood and help prevent "sitting diseases" such as obesity and poor cardiovascular fitness.

Also, eat healthy foods, stick to a good sleep schedule, and connect with others to ward off loneliness. All of these healthy habits will boost your immune system and your state of mind.

6. Pregnancy risks

Some seers have predicted a coronavirus baby boom. If you and your partner do not want to get pregnant, make sure you have a supply of condoms or another method of birth control on hand.

Dangers from Living Companions

While outside the scope of this essay, I would just like to mention some extreme safety hazards that you might face from others in your home. I'll offer a quick list, followed by one or more resources:

- *Partner abuse.* The National Domestic Violence Hotline is open 24/7: 1-800-799-SAFE or text LOVEIS to 22522. Or just call 911.
- *Child abuse.* 1-800-4-A-CHILD (1-800-422-4453) is the National Child Abuse Hotline, open 24/7. Their text number is 1-800-422-4453.
- *Alcohol or drug abuse.* The New York Times published a comprehensive list of online resources for those who struggle with substance abuse and their friends and family: https://www.nytimes.com/2020/03/26/health/coronavirus-sobriety-online-help.html?searchResultPosition=1

- *National Suicide Hotline*: 1-800-273-8255.

Sadly, all of these dangers appear to be on the increase now that people are trapped at home. What you can do: Put the necessary phone numbers in your contact list now. If you can, discuss your situation with a trusted friend, relative, or an expert on the hotline.

It's Safe to Say …

Many good people ask what they can do to help others during this crisis. The answer to that question might be: First do no harm…to yourself. Second, to help others, stay at home. With just a few simple adjustments, your home can become a safer space. And by keeping yourself safe and healthy, you don't add to the load on an already overwhelmed health care system.

There are real dangers out there, dangers that you can't control. But one of the quickest ways to reduce stress is to control what you can—and that could be the safety of your living space.

© Meg Selig. Posted on psychologytoday.com, 4.3.2020.

References

Casden, S. "Do Not Stand on That Chair." Slate.com: March 26, 2020. (I also highly recommend Casden's book, *Careful*.)

Schlanger, Z. "Now is the time to take care of your lungs. Here's how." *New York Times*: March 27, 2020.

Silverman, L. (2014) "Broken Hips: Preventing a Fall Can Save Your Life," NPR.

OTHER VOICES:
Safe, Healthy, and Wise

"At the age of 18, I made up my mind to never have another bad day in my life. I dove into an endless sea of gratitude from which I've never emerged."

—Patch Adams

"Of all the self-fulfilling prophecies in our culture the assumption that aging means decline and poor health is probably the deadliest."

—Marilyn Ferguson

"I have chosen to be happy. It's good for my health."

—Voltaire

"Laugh and your cells laugh with you."

—Cari Corbet-Owen

"(G)rowing into your future with health and grace and beauty doesn't have to take all your time. It rather requires a dedication to caring for yourself as if you were rare and precious, which you are, and regarding all life around you as equally so, which it is."

—Victoria Moran

PART IV
PATHWAYS TO SUCCESSFUL AGING

CHAPTER 24

STILL GROWING: THREE PATHWAYS TO SUCCESSFUL AGING

> "Those of us living today have been handed a remarkable gift with no strings attached: an extra thirty years of life for the average person... What are we going to do with super-sized lives?"
> — Dr. Laura Carstensen

The Challenge

By 2050, 10% of the U.S. population will be 90 or older, according to the Census Bureau. What are we going to do with our "super-sized lives?"

That is the question posed by Laura Carstensen, an expert on aging, in her book, *A Long Bright Future*.

Assuming the coronavirus crisis and its aftermath do not significantly change the trajectory of human longevity (and, writing these words in the midst of it, I worry about that), those who retire at age 65 could easily have 20-30 more years of active life. How can you make the most of those precious

30 years? Whether retired or not, how could you ensure that your older years are happy and healthy ones?

The term "successful aging" is often used to describe an aging process that is fulfilling, happy, and healthy for as long as possible. While experts differ, most would agree that the key elements of successful aging are "life satisfaction, longevity, freedom from disability, mastery and growth, active engagement with life, and independence," according to aging expert Harry Moody.

In this post, I'll describe three pathways to successful aging. I've mapped these routes in part from research, in part from my personal experience and that of others my age. A given person could follow these paths in sequence or go back and forth among them. In a way, we are always on all three paths, at any age, at any given time.

But—and this is a big *but*—all three concepts of successful aging depend heavily on another set of factors, factors described in the last section.

Path 1: Youthful Aging, a.k.a. Active Aging

The motto for this path could be, "Forever young." Although many of us older people would shudder at the idea of reliving our youth, the idea of looking and feeling perpetually youthful is appealing. There are even some healthy and realistic ways to do it, as I discuss in the chapter, "How Far Can You Turn Back the Clock on Aging?" At its best, this path is characterized by dedicated self-care—preventing diseases of aging through exercise, healthy eating, stress reduction, good relationships, and other healthy habits. When focused on healthful behaviors, followers of this path can frequently avoid many diseases of aging and stay stronger longer.

Sometimes the good intentions of the Youthful Agers get hijacked by the "anti-aging industrial complex," as described by Susan Douglas in her book, *In Our Prime*. According to Douglas, beauty companies and their advertisers urge older people, especially women, to use their "age-defying" products and do the impossible: Never grow or look old. When looking older is somehow suspect—you aren't trying hard enough!—the anti-aging attitude can easily slip into ageism, as Douglas points out.

The youthful aging path has a huge upside. With luck, you may feel as young as ever. Plus, youthful, active older people help dent the stereotypes about aging, broadening everyone's idea of what "old" really is. That process is "age-defying" in the best sense of the word.

Path 2: Productive Aging

Like Path 1, this aging pathway focuses on sustaining health and vitality but broadens the idea of successful aging to include "productive aging." Productive aging emphasizes an active search for a purposeful life as one ages. A meaningful life can involve contributing to society through work, grandparenting, volunteer work, a legacy project, or helping others.

Many on this path might boast that their motto is, "Never retire." Certainly, productive aging can involve the goal of continuing to earn money, whether to build up savings, contribute to the next generation, or shore up the ability to live independently. Let's face it—money can help seniors stay independent and buy some of the services they may need—housekeeping, gardening, and transportation, among others.

Youthful aging and productive aging crisscross in that they share the idea that "A good old age...is just an old age with minimum sickness or frailty, as much like youth or midlife as possible," as Moody puts it. For older people who desire to pursue meaningful career or retirement goals, good health and energy are essential. If you are an athlete, leader, teacher, or anyone with an ambitious goal, you need stamina and grit to keep going.

With luck, good genes, and good habits, many older people could have a "healthspan" that is almost identical to their lifespan. However, most of us will find that our health status will change, whether dramatically or in small steps. And that's where the third path comes in.

Path 3: Conscious Aging

Eventually, most of us can no longer postpone decline but must adapt to it. "Conscious aging"* refers to the deliberate choice to tap into creativity, inner strength, spirituality, and mindfulness to meet life's demands despite losses of strength, mobility, and productivity. Creatively compensating for those losses can become one marker of successful aging on this third pathway.

There are at least three helpful ways to age consciously. One way is behavioral—through figuring out adequate substitutes for activities that various limitations have rendered impossible. In the realm of exercise, for example, a person might walk instead of jog or run. In the realm of social contribution, an older person might offer emotional support to children and grandchildren, even though he can no longer provide direct care.

A second way to age consciously is by becoming more mindful of the small details of daily life and appreciating them. Coffee with a friend, the light at dusk, a shapely vase, flowers, trees— older people learn to savor all these small pleasures. While not exclusive to the conscious aging path by any means, the ability to enjoy life's small pleasures is a great comfort in later years.

A third way to age consciously is by changing one's inner attitude. Viktor Frankl, who wrote about his survival in the concentration camps of Nazi Germany, famously wrote: "Everything can be taken from a man but one thing: the last of the human freedoms—to choose one's attitude in any given set of circumstances, to choose one's own way."

How do the oldest old cultivate attitudes that promote coping and even growth? As Moody puts it, "Personal meaning is sustained through inner resources permitting continued growth even in the face of loss, pain, and physical decline." "Inner resources" could include various acts of introspection. Either alone or with help, elders might conduct a "life review," allowing them to relive and discover new meaning in the events of their life. They could make an inner decision to become role models who demonstrate bravery in the face of suffering and death. They could focus on positive emotions such as gratitude that enable them to face the future with some degree of equanimity.

What Makes All Three Types of Successful Aging Possible?

American culture tends to place a premium on self-reliance, individualism, and hard work. These traits can indeed promote successful aging.

But, as numerous experts point out, notably Louise Aronson in her prize-winning book *Elderhood,* the journey through old age must rest as well on a foundation of societal support. This support should begin at infancy and continue through adulthood and old age. Longevity and wellness for seniors is only possible if we can prevent and cure diseases throughout the life cycle, encourage and teach healthy behaviors, and provide access to medical, mental health, and dental care.

Besides social services and healthcare, specific resources for seniors could also include: assistive devices, such as hearing aids and glasses (not currently reimbursed by Medicare); help and compensation for caregivers; excellent rehab facilities, nursing homes, and hospice care; physical and occupational therapy; an end to age discrimination in employment; pensions and other financial resources; and a reasonable retirement age. Our social safety net must be mended and extended so that these benefits are available to all.

Otherwise, the "Golden Years" will be tarnished by poverty and ill health, except for the very wealthiest among us. And that is a shame when successful aging could easily be within the reach of all.

© Meg Selig. First published on PsychologyToday.com, May 17, 2020.

The phrase "conscious aging" can be traced at least as far back as a 1992 book by that name, authored by Ram Dass.

References

Harry R. Moody, "From Successful Aging to Conscious Aging," in Wykle, M.L. et al, *Successful Aging Through the Life Span* (2005), NY: Springer Publishing. I highly recommend this remarkable essay!

Carstensen, L. (2011) *A Long Bright Future: Happiness, Health, and Financial Security in an Age of Increased Longevity*. NY: PublicAffairsT.

Douglas, S. J. (2020). *In Our Prime: How Older Women Are Reinventing the Road Ahead*. NY: WW Norton.

Aronson, L. (2019) *Elderhood: Redefining Aging, Transforming Medicine, Reimagining Life*. NY: Bloomsbury Publishing.

CHAPTER 25

SEVEN 'PILLS' FOR HEALTH, LONG LIFE, AND HAPPINESS

Mind, body, and spirit benefit from these seven "pills." Don't worry, these pills go down easy!

These "Pills" Are Pillars of Your Health

Do you ever wish you could just take a few pills and suddenly blossom into your best health? You can!

Well, okay, these "pills" aren't exactly the kind that you swallow in a gulp, and that's that. They are *practices* rather than, say, a vitamin pill. Still, all these recommendations are easy to follow and can fit snugly into your day. Moreover, they are completely natural and have zero to few negative side effects. And these seven pills are not fads: Overwhelming amounts of scientific research tell us that these pills are—forgive the pun—pillars of human health.

The seven pills are not "bitter pills," the distasteful but necessary things or people that we sometimes have to tolerate in our lives. These pills go down easy, especially if you creatively adapt them to your own needs.

Some of these pills will not surprise you. But are you aware of numbers 1, 4, 5, and 7 below? Check out all seven, including proposed Pill #8. Pill #8 is the only one that might be considered controversial.

1. The Nature Pill

Numerous studies have demonstrated that a "Nature Pill," a.k.a., "Vitamin N," such as hiking in a natural area or even strolling briefly outside, is an excellent stress reliever. While some stress motivates you to meet the challenges of life, *excess* stress causes the body to produce the stress hormone cortisol. Cortisol is strongly linked to health problems such as heart disease, depression, sleep issues, dementia, and many more.

Smallest Dose: Even tiny doses of nature—such as having green plants in your office or looking out the window at the trees—seem to cause a measurable drop in cortisol, according to many studies.

Minimum Dose: A recent study found that a "dose" of nature of only 20 minutes was enough to lower cortisol to a healthier level. In this study, participants decided for themselves what kind of experience made them feel that they'd been in contact with nature. Then, using saliva samples to check cortisol, researchers found that participants who took a 20-minute Nature Pill lowered their cortisol levels significantly regardless of whether they sat or moved about in a natural area. Park bench, anyone?

Ideal Dose: Researchers discovered that 30 minutes immersed in nature was even better than 20 for lowering cortisol levels; after that, benefits continued but were negligible.

2. The Exercise Pill

This amazing pill can...(take a deep breath—a long list is coming)...maintain muscle strength, prevent lower back pain, boost the immune system, strengthen bones, elevate mood, ease mild depression, lower blood pressure, reduce diabetes risk, strengthen bones, promote healthier brain functioning, keep you at a healthy weight, and even reverse some aspects of aging, among countless other benefits. Every day amazing new discoveries about the health power of exercise attest to the potency of this pill.

You may worry that a regular exercise regimen is just too hard for you right now. No problem! Exercise pills come in small, medium, and large, and almost any dose is helpful.

Minimum Dose: Many research studies have come to the same conclusion: Even small amounts of exercise—aka, "exercise snacks"—can have powerful positive effects on mind and body. The trick seems to be to move around for about five minutes every hour; this small "bite" of exercise can reduce your risk of "sitting diseases" such as diabetes, obesity, heart disease, and some cancers.

Ideal Dose: For moderate exercisers, the World Health Organization recommends 150 minutes of exercise per week (say, 30 minutes/day, 5 days/week) for adults. Your ideal dose will depend on your exercise goals. If your goal is to run a marathon, you will need a large dose of exercise.

Note: The Nature Pill and the Exercise Pill make beautiful health music together.

3. The Mediterranean Pill

A Mediterranean diet has been linked in research to better brain health, reduced risk of heart attacks, strokes, cancer, and Alzheimer's, as well as reduced mortality overall. To follow this healthy eating plan, eat mostly fruits, vegetables and other plant-based foods such as legumes, nuts, and whole grains; reduce use of saturated fats like butter and replace them with healthy fats like canola and olive oil; limit added sugars; use herbs instead of salt; eat moderate amounts of chicken and fish; and limit red meat. And don't forget the tea and coffee: They, too, seem to promote better brainpower.

I like the Mediterranean eating plan because no foods are forbidden. You just have to reduce your intake of unhealthy foods. This is difficult but possible.

Disease-reversing dose: Those who suffer from certain chronic diseases such as heart disease or diabetes may want to follow the Ornish diet (named after Dr. Dean Ornish, the creator of the diet.) This plant-based diet, along with exercise, stress management, and social support, has been shown in many studies to reverse even intractable conditions such as severe coronary heart disease, type 2 diabetes, elevated blood pressure, high cholesterol, and obesity.

4. The Stress-Management Pill

Excess stress and chronic stress can cause multiple problems due to the impact of the stress hormone cortisol on your body. For instance, stress can raise your risk of heart problems. Stress also can cause mental health problems, fatigue, and inflammation.

"Reframing can be as simple as telling yourself that you face a "challenge," not a "problem."

Everyone needs a daily stress reduction technique. Possibilities include some combination of the following: deep breathing, yoga, meditation, exercise, reframing (see below), or the Nature Pill.

Part of the harm of stress comes from our perception that stress is overwhelming. So reframing the issues that you face can be an essential quick-fix solution. "Reframing" is simply a different way of looking at a person, situation, or relationship. A reframe can be as simple as telling yourself that you face a "challenge," not a "problem."

A major superpower of stress reduction techniques is that they lower blood pressure. In fact, one study found that meditation helped 40 out of 60 patients lower their blood pressure enough to reduce some medications.

Smallest dose: One deep breath. Amazingly, just one deep breath can turn down your flight-or-fight response and give you an ounce more of calm. In addition, learning to pause in the midst of a conflict or a stressful situation to take a few deep breaths can help you make better decisions, preserve your relationships, and protect your health by reducing cortisol.

Recommended minimum dose: Just 10 minutes of stress reduction per day is helpful, according to the *Harvard Health Letter*.

Creativity and problem-solving dose: Take a 20-minute break. During the break, your brain will release chemicals that counter the stress response, enabling you to shift into a more creative mode of thinking.

5. The Love and Relationships Pill

In our individualistic society, we often forget the importance of social support. But countless studies have shown that good relationships promote health, happiness, and longevity, and reduce the incidence of depression, loneliness, and early death. In one such study, the Harvard Study of Adult Development, over 700 men were followed from 1938 to the present (about 60 remain from the original 724). Researchers found a strong association between close relationships, happiness, longevity, and health.

> "Happiness is love. Full stop."
> —Dr. George Vailliant, director of the Harvard Study of Adult Development.

Why? Safe and supportive social relationships help calm our stress-response system. Lower levels of stress hormones (cortisol again) mean less wear and tear on the brain and body, longer life, and more joy in daily living. In fact, neuropsychologist Louis Cozolino, the author of *Timeless: Nature's Formula for Health and Longevity*, asserts that, "People who lead extraordinarily long lives are those who have maintained close ties to others."

Dose: May vary with your personality type. The general idea is: Find good people, stay connected with them, and join support groups. Maintain your social safety net by keeping up with friends, colleagues, and relatives, and by mending frayed relationships when you can. Love others.

6. The Sleep Pill

Shakespeare was right; sleep does knit up the "raveled sleeve of care." That's because lack of sleep increases cortisol, the problematic stress hormone mentioned several times above. It also leads to unhealthy inflammation, and, of course, contributes to physical and mental fatigue. In general, longer sleep duration is associated with greater longevity. Specifically, six hours of sleep or less is linked to shorter telomeres (those caps on your chromosomes that protect them from deteriorating), while nine hours of sleep is associated with longer telomeres.

Dose: Most health professionals recommend that adults get 7-9 hours of sleep each night.

7. The Gratitude Pill

Gratitude, along with its cousins, happiness, and purpose, can provide a powerful infusion of emotional health for most people. Numerous studies suggest that a "gratitude practice," such as the iconic "Three Good Things" exercise, is a powerful contributor to happiness. The exercise is simple: For five minutes at the end of the day, think or write about three good things that happened to you and whether those good things were due to luck or to something you did. Doing this exercise for just one week raised participants' happiness levels for six months. Six months! The "gratitude attitude" has been linked in research to other positive emotions, such as joy, enthusiasm, and optimism, not just to happiness, and even seems to boost self-control.

Minimum Dose: Five minutes. Five minutes of a gratitude practice daily for just one week can boost your happiness level for six months...and maybe get you into a healthy habit that lasts for a lifetime.

The Eighth Pill: Healthcare for All?

With exceptions, the seven practices above are within the control of most people. It's wonderful that we can choose to prevent certain diseases or enhance our health and vitality with such simple activities.

But even though we may work hard at keeping fit and healthy, our genes, bad luck, and the aging process can trip up our efforts. In addition, people may be in the pink of good health and still become victims of accidents, diseases, and personal tragedies. It is at such times that we may realize that excellent health is not just a matter of individual effort but of protective social resources.

That's why we need an eighth pill for health and happiness—a Healthcare-for-All Pill. Without it, many people cannot hope to live a long, fulfilling, and happy life, because they must scramble for basic medical and dental necessities, often in times of personal crisis and confusion. Moreover, those without health insurance live a stressful life, lacking a basic pillar of psychological safety—a healthcare safety net.

The United States does not score near the top in global surveys of longevity, health, and happiness. While these surveys must be taken with grains of salt and a little perspective, in general, they tell a disturbing story of American inadequacy in these areas. To summarize: In longevity, the United States ranks 31 in a 2015 World Health Organization survey. In the 2018 United Nations World Happiness Report, the U.S. ranks 18. On the Bloomberg Global Health Index of 2019, the U.S. does not even make the top 25.

The trends are not positive, but they could be reversed with a sustained national effort.

Take Those Pills!

Someone once asked my late father what he usually had for breakfast. In his late 80's at the time, he replied, "Cereal, OJ, coffee, and a handful of pills." This humorous reply was laced with a touch of sarcasm. However, I don't think he would have minded taking the seven pills above. In fact, he did take most of them, which is probably why he lived to 91, healthy, with all his faculties, and always interested in those he loved.

© Meg Selig, Posted on psychologytoday.com, Apr 30, 2019.

References

"Stressed? Take a 20-minute 'nature pill,'" *ScienceDaily* (2019): https://www.sciencedaily.com/releases/2019/04/190404074915.htm

Mediterranean diet: A heart-healthy eating plan, Mayo Clinic, 2019: https://www.mayoclinic.org/healthy-lifestyle/nutrition-and-healthy-eating/in-depth/mediterranean-diet/art-20047801

The Harvard Health Letter, April 2019: "In fact, the Ornish Lifestyle Medicine program (www.ornish.com) is so well accepted that Medicare has been reimbursing participants since 2010."

Lower blood pressure. Aubrey, A., "High Stress Drives Up Your Risk Of A Heart Attack. Here's How To Chill Out." NPR, April 14, 2019.

10 minutes of stress reduction. "Losing steam? Avoid these energy zappers," *Harvard Health Letter*, April 2019.

Evans, K. "Why Relationships are the Key to Longevity," 9.17.2018, mindful.org.

Sleep and telomeres. Starkweather, A.R. "An Integrative Review of Factors Associated with Telomere Length and Implications for Biobehavioral Research," July 2014: https://www.ncbi.nlm.nih.gov/pmc/articles/PMC4112289/

CHAPTER 26

SEEKING THE FOUNTAIN OF YOUTH? 10 TIPS TO REVERSE AGING

Youthful aging, anyone? These 10 simple strategies can slow, or even reverse, the aging process.

How Far Can You Turn Back the Clock on Aging?

In 2018 a 69-year-old man from the Netherlands applied to change his birth date to one that would make him 20 years younger. It turned out that he was having trouble finding prospective partners on Internet dating sites. He felt that being able to say he was only 49 would help his mating search. The court turned him down.

When I first read about this unusual request, I said to myself, "I think I know why this guy has so much trouble finding dates, and it has nothing to do with his age."

But then I reprimanded myself for being "judge-y." After all, what older person—including me—does not want to come across as younger? And what single person looking for love does not want to put their best foot—and face—forward?

As I continued to ponder this problem, I realized that there are a number of ways that older people can legitimately hold back the tide of aging—not by changing their birth date, but by changing their habits and by taking advantage of technology and science.

Of course, there are plenty of **cosmetic solutions** that can improve someone's looks. Many are easy and relatively harmless, such as coloring your hair, using makeup, and whitening your teeth. There are also **attitude solutions** to the challenges of growing older. You can decide to accept the aging process and "grow old gracefully." And whatever your age, you can be "young at heart."

This essay, however, will focus on actual **age-reversing solutions** that have either been extensively researched or that show significant promise of effectiveness. By "age-reversing," I mean activities, treatments, or therapies that can slow or even reverse biological aging. Specifically, many actions on the list below act at the cellular level by repairing and lengthening telomeres—those caps at the ends of chromosomes that shorten as a result of aging—thereby reducing your DNA age (a.k.a, your "biologic age"). Other items on the list repair, replace, or regenerate aging body parts.

I must admit that it is sometimes difficult to distinguish between actions that reverse aging and those that lengthen the life span, improve general health, or increase well-being. You will notice some gray areas. Also, I've excluded any actions that are too expensive, high-risk, or cause extensive suffering. You will not see facelifts on the list because they are expensive and, in some cases, dangerous. (However, I see nothing wrong with these if you can afford it and feel that the risks are worth it for you.) The items below are simple, low-cost, and low-tech, yet can bring about a youthful transformation.

(Caution: While science-based, some results that I describe below are based on small studies. Others describe correlation not causation. Consult your health professional for medical advice tailored to your health conditions and situation.)

10 Easy Ways to Become Younger

1. Use retinoids.

Retinoids, including the most well-known brand, Retin-A, are topical skin lotions that perform a multitude of miracles, including reducing skin aging. They treat acne, lighten age spots, reduce wrinkles, and firm the skin. These wonder drugs can even soften rough patches of skin and lighten brown spots caused by sun exposure.

Retinoids work at the DNA level, increasing the skin's production of collagen (the substance that keeps the skin firm), stimulating the growth of new blood vessels (a process which improves skin tone), and speeding the turnover of surface skin cells so new healthy cells can take their place. Retinoids fix so many skin problems with so few side-effects that one dermatologist quoted on WebMD said, "I recommend retinoids to everybody." (Naturally, you should consult with your dermatologist about if and how to use retinoids in your case.)

2. Use sunscreen.

Sunscreen is a valuable anti-aging tool. It prevents premature skin aging, protects your skin from harmful UVA (aging) rays and UVB (burning) rays, and guards against many skin cancers. If you are using a retinoid lotion at night, it is essential to apply sunscreen daily, as retinoids cause susceptibility to sunburn. And you know that tanning beds increase your risk of skin cancers, right?

3. Exercise reverses aging, especially this kind of exercise.

You may already know that exercise possesses magical powers to prevent diseases and to promote both physical and mental health. Now for something even more magical: Exercise may actually reverse certain types of aging.

In a study from 2018, researchers studied a small group of people in their 70's who had exercised regularly over their life span. They had the cardiovascular health of those 30 years younger. These lifelong exercisers were also compared to active young people in their 20's. While the elders did not possess the aerobic capacity of the younger exercisers, the muscles of the older exercisers did resemble those of young people, even down to the number of capillaries and enzymes.

Added to these results, a study from 2017, reported by Mike Zimmerman in the *AARP Bulletin*, compared telomere length in sedentary and active adults. The researchers found that exercisers had a nine-year aging advantage.

And the one kind of exercise that appears to be particularly helpful? High-Intensity Interval Training (HIIT) slows aging and increases telomere length, according to Zimmerman. Basically, HITT programs involve alternating easy to moderate intensity exercise with short bursts of high-intensity exercise. My modified HIIT exercise: walk the sidewalks, jog the streets—or at least, a few of them.

4. Reverse decline in muscle strength with this simple exercise program.

"Sarcopenia" means a decline in skeletal muscle strength as a result of aging. (Sarcopenia is to muscles what osteopenia is to bones.) Loss of muscle mass can lead to falls, inability to perform simple daily tasks, and loss of independence. Many doctors do not even warn their patients about the debilitating effects of this condition, according to *New York Times* health writer Jane Brody.

But sarcopenia can be reversed at any—and I mean *any*—age! Brody writes that, "No matter how old or out of shape you are, you can restore much of the strength you already lost.... research documenting the ability to reverse the losses of sarcopenia—even among nursing home residents in their

90s—has been in the medical literature for 30 years, and the time is long overdue to act on it."

What works? Strength training, a.k.a weight lifting or resistance training. You can use free weights, bands, or machines, gradually increasing the degree of difficulty.

5. Sex may be good for your telomeres.

A very small but suggestive 2017 study of 129 women found that those women who'd had sex with their long-term partner during the week had significantly longer telomeres and more telomerase (the enzyme that stimulates the growth of telomeres) than those women who did not.

Surprisingly, telomere length was not associated with factors like relationship satisfaction or stress. But which came first—healthier women or partner sex? The researchers acknowledged that healthier women with longer telomeres could be more interested in sex. Still, the results are intriguing.

6. Take advantage of ED medications.

And speaking of sex, you could also consider medications for erectile dysfunction (ED).

A colleague of mine worked for the Masters and Johnson Institute for many years. If a man had erectile dysfunction, the therapists at the Institute recommended that the couple do a series of "sensate focus" exercises over a period of weeks. "Now I would just recommend Viagra," he said. "Let's face it: It's a medical miracle."

Of course, the decision to use any ED medication should be made as a couple. And ED meds are not a cure for relationship issues. Couples with problems should consider seeing a couples therapist.

Also, not every man is an appropriate candidate for ED drugs. See your doctor for details.

7. Sleep well.

In general, longer sleep duration is associated with longer telomeres. Specifically, six hours of sleep or less is linked to shorter telomeres, while nine hours of sleep is associated with longer telomeres. (Results vary depending on age and other factors.) Most health professionals recommend getting 7-9 hours of sleep each night.

8. Look into cataract surgery.

I am including this medical procedure because it is outpatient, very low-risk, and covered by Medicare and other insurance plans. This amazing surgery involves replacing the cloudy, aging lenses of the eye with artificial lenses that restore youthful sight. "Was blind but now I see" accurately describes the experience of some patients. My own experience was more complicated, but I am clearly better off than before.

9. Meditate: It's exercise for the mind.

Sara Lazar, a neuroscientist with Harvard Medical School, has studied the effects of meditation on the brain. Her 2005 study showed that regular meditators had more gray matter in the prefrontal cortex (PFC), the executive area of the brain. Moreover, 50-year-old meditators had as much gray matter as 25-year-olds, leading Lazar to hypothesize that meditation could reverse or slow the natural age-related atrophy of the brain.

Another one of her studies indicated that just eight weeks of regular meditation practice could thicken the memory part of the brain, the hippocampus, and reduce the stress reaction in the amygdala, the flight-or-flight area.

In 2014, Lazar and colleagues reviewed 12 studies about meditation and cognitive decline, concluding that "meditation techniques may be able to offset age-related cognitive decline and perhaps even increase cognitive capabilities in older adults."

10. Good relationships promote health, happiness, and longevity.

The Harvard Study of Adult Development has followed over 700 men since 1938. The results have consistently shown that good social relationships promote physical and mental health, provide a buffer against loneliness, increase longevity, and foster happiness. The Harvard Nurses' Health Study found similar results for women.

Why? Safe and supportive social relationships help calm our stress-response system, according to health writer Karin Evan. Lower levels of stress hormones such as cortisol mean less wear and tear on the brain and body, longer life, and more joy in daily living.

Other Possible Age-Reversers

People who want to live long and prosper could take advantage of other activities that are linked to a more youthful old age. For example, research shows that older people who have a purpose in life tend to sleep better, have better brain health, and feel happier. A Mediterranean diet has been linked in some research to better brain health. The decision to adopt better posture when standing, sitting, or moving may not change your DNA, but good posture is an easy way to broadcast youth and vitality, help you breathe better, and protect your spine, shoulders, and neck.

So, don't try to change your birth date with an official piece of paper. Instead, focus on choices that will promote physical and mental health, vitality, connection with others, and longevity. Although time and trouble will happen to us all, we can make numerous positive changes in both our actions and attitudes, as well as learn to accept what we cannot change.

Note: This blog emerged out of an email exchange between my sister Kate Kimelman and me. Thanks for your input, Kate! Kate is an editor in the Bay Area.

© Meg Selig. Posted Feb 28, 2019, on psychologytoday.com.

References

Domonoske, C. "69-Year-Old Dutch Man Seeks to Change His Legal Age to 49," 11.8.2018, NPR.

Zimmerman, M. "Ways to Add Healthy Years to Your Life," *AARP Bulletin*, Jan/Feb 2019, p. 10-16.

Edgar, J. "Retinoids for Anti-Aging Skin," 2011, WebMd.

Brody, J. "Preventing Muscle Loss as We Age," Sept., 2018, *New York Times*.

Evans, K. "Why Relationships Are the Key to Longevity," mindful.org.

Dolan, E.W. "Study finds sexual intimacy is associated with longer telomere length in women," July, 2017, psypost.org.

Starkweather, A. et al, "An Integrative Review of Factors Associated With Telomere Length," https://www.ncbi.nlm.nih.gov/pmc/articles/PMC4112289/, Nurs Res. 2014 Jan-Feb; 63(1): 36–50.

Alderman, L. "The Surprising Benefits of Meditation for Brain Health," considerable.com.

"Posture." https://newsinhealth.nih.gov/2017/08/getting-it-straight

One Small Spark:

A Hairy Story

I have mixed feelings about my silvering hair. On the one hand, I would like to accept my appearance as it is. To do otherwise would be a type of internalized ageism. On the other hand, I would like to look as attractive and youthful as possible for as long as possible. Looking good lifts morale.

One day I approached Roger, my hairdresser of forty years. "I'm thinking about dyeing my hair," I told him.

"We do not use the word 'dye,' " he explained with authority. "You do not 'dye' your hair. You "color" your hair. Then you die."

Okay, that helps.

OTHER VOICES:
Youthful Aging

"There is a fountain of youth: it is your mind, your talents, the creativity you bring to your life and the lives of people you love. When you learn to tap this source, you will truly have defeated age."

—Sophia Loren

"Exercise is roughly the only equivalent of a fountain of youth that exists today, and it's free to everyone."

—S. Jay Olshansky, Gerontologist

"You are never too old to look younger."

—Mae West

"Inside every older person is a younger person wondering what happened."

—Jennifer Yane

"If you don't make time for exercise, you'll probably have to make time for illness."

—Robin Sharma

"Those who love deeply never grow old: They may die of old age, but they die young."

—Ben Franklin

CHAPTER 27

THE COMMON MEDICAL PROBLEM THAT UPENDED MY ENTIRE LIFE: A PERSONAL ESSAY

"PF was the first condition to threaten my mobility and therefore my sense of freedom and autonomy."

As a dedicated exerciser, healthy eater, meditator, and health writer, I never dreamed that the Achilles' heel in my health life would be...my Achilles' heel.

When I was 74, I developed a severe case of plantar fasciitis (PF)—heel pain—in my left foot. {*Plantar fasciitis* (PLAN-tur fas-e-I-tis) involves inflammation of a thick band of tissue, the *plantar fascia*, which runs lengthwise from your Achilles heel along the bottom of your foot down to your toes.}

I'd had PF before. Thirty years ago, I'd visited an orthopedist because of stabbing pains in my left foot. The orthopedist supplied me with the PF diagnosis and gave me a set of simple stretching exercises to do three times a day when it flared up. Problem solved.

Now it was a different story. Again my left foot was involved, but this time I felt intense pain with every step. The old exercises lost their power to heal. I found myself limping, unable to stride forward with my usual speed and confidence.

I decided to return to the helpful orthopedist. Because I was now considered a new patient, he did not have an available appointment for six months, so I signed up with his nurse practitioner. She was a grim-faced woman who gave me six exercises to do five times a day, a giant night splint to stretch my arch while I slept, instructions for shoe-buying, and a physical therapy referral. She warned me that unless I followed this regimen, I would be doomed to a life of heel pain.

I thought of her as "the plantar fascist." But she was thorough, I'll grant her that.

Disgracefully, I never could quite motivate myself to do all the exercises required each day, but I did most of them. I went to physical therapy where I was assigned even more exercises. I tried laser light therapy. I bought better shoes. I slept with the boot on.

Nothing worked, and I was exhausted.

• • •

I tried to see this problem in perspective. In the great scheme of things, plantar fasciitis is not on the same scale as cancer, heart disease, ALS, or diabetes. In the small scheme of things, however, PF was an insidious and painful condition, affecting my mood, my energy, and my mobility. It took me a while to realize that while I was more fortunate than others, I was still in pain and deserved some self-compassion.

I feel badly when I whine about pain, but a stronger friend with a similar foot problem said: "This whole thing has been worse than any surgery I've ever had, or even breast cancer for that matter."

PF was not the first chronic illness to come into my life. I had chronic migraines and a host of other minor health problems. But PF was the only condition to threaten my mobility and therefore my sense of independence. As I stumbled about, I began to feel old for the first time.

Because of PF, my entire life changed. I had always loved to walk and for years had walked for 30 minutes almost daily. I had also followed every other sensible recommendation about physical activity—don't sit for too long, use the stairs, find reasons to move, lift weights twice a week.

What do you do when you are a walker, and you can't walk? When you understand the power of exercise, but you can't be on your feet? When just standing up becomes an ordeal?

• • •

First, I dumped the plantar fascist and found a decent podiatrist. She listened to a recital of my attempts to cure the PF and announced, "OK, you've tried a lot of things, so I'm not messing around with you. You need orthotics and a cortisone shot." Two cortisone shots and one pair of orthotics later, and my foot was almost back to normal.

Then, I found creative ways to adapt. Because I didn't want to push my luck, I had to consider various options to my beloved 30-minute walks. As a confirmed land mammal, I refused to become a swimmer. But I discovered I could take 20-minute walks without suffering later. To protect my feet further, I alternated walking with non-walking exercise, like lifting weights or cycling. I became a regular on the exercise bike at my physical therapist's office. I'm not crazy about cycling, but I enjoyed chatting with the other patients and discovered that most of them had more severe physical problems than I.

Now, approximately one year later, my foot is better. I can even walk for 30 minutes if I don't do it too often.

The PF is always lurking in the background, however, ready to strike again.

• • •

During the eight-month period of coping with PF, I had many down moments. During one especially discouraging episode, I decided to see a therapist. He said something I will never forget: "Well, for most of your life, your feet took care of you. Now it's your turn to take care of your feet."

And that's what I'm doing now.

I bathe my feet with lotion and gently massage them before I put on my socks each morning. I don't stress them with needless standing. When the COVID crisis is over, I will treat them to a pedicure. With luck, I've got a lot of living to do, and, if possible, I want to do it on my own two feet.

© Meg Selig, 2020.

CHAPTER 28

HOW TO BOUNCE BACK FROM AGING CHALLENGES

Both joy and despair will be part of the aging journey.

The Case of the Disappearing Groceries

The other day I was at the supermarket, happily putting some of my favorite goodies into my cart. But as I wheeled toward the cashier, items began mysteriously disappearing. I looked around to catch the thief in the act but saw no one. By the time I got to the check-out line, every single item I had chosen had vanished. My cart was now empty.

I was livid. I stormed at the clerk: "What kind of a place is this? All of my groceries have disappeared! Every single thing is gone!"

I was so furious that I woke myself up.

The Challenges of Aging

Sometimes the unconscious mind really nails it. Yes, what kind of place *is* this? This year, as I approached yet another landmark birthday, I had been assailed by numerous minor chronic illnesses and conditions—death by a thousand cuts, as I described it to myself. One of these conditions, an intractable eight-months-long case of heel pain (plantar fasciitis), was causing me to hurt literally with every step, preventing me from moving about with ease and from engaging in my favorite exercise—walking.

But while the unconscious mind may have a direct pipeline to one's current emotional life, it lacks perspective. It was not true that all the good things in my life were vanishing one at a time, and that all that remained was to "check out." My physical ailments were annoying, painful, and inconvenient, but none were life-threatening. I had every reason to believe that the heel pain might go into remission at some point. Most importantly, I had an abundance of blessings in my life—a wonderful partner and family, interesting work, friends, and numerous small pleasures.

Still, the dream reflected a certain kind of truth—that I was now facing the realities of aging. It was not a pleasant truth. At times I felt stabs of depression and despair. I realized I needed to find a more hopeful perspective, one that could keep me optimistic, stop the needless catastrophizing, and help me cope with my "new normal."

> "Many of us have learned that happiness is a skill and a choice. We don't need to look at our horoscopes to know how our day will go. We know how to create a good day."
> — Mary Pipher

14 Ways to Bounce Back from Aging Challenges

I began experimenting with a variety of strategies, some science-backed, some idiosyncratic. I'd like to emphasize that while these strategies worked for me in varying degrees, everyone is different. Still, my hope is that anyone in a similar situation to mine could adapt these strategies to their own aging or health challenges, at whatever age they might be. Here is what I learned and re-learned:

1. *First and foremost, give yourself the gift of self-compassion.* Self-compassion will prevent you from adding self-criticism to your burden of suffering. For example, because my problems are small in comparison to those with more serious health conditions, I tend to discount them. I've even caught my critical inner voice labeling myself a "wimp." This is not helpful! Pain hurts, even if the pain of another may be greater. If "self-compassion" seems like an abstract idea to you, try this mantra from author Kristin Neff's book *Self-Compassion*: "This is a moment of suffering. Suffering is part of life. May I be kind to me in this moment. May I give myself the compassion I need." For quick access to this wisdom, memorize it.

2. *Look your best.* Some people would condemn such advice as shallow or vain. Maybe it is. But vanity can be a great motivator for healthy change. And looking good can raise morale and self-esteem. "When you put in the effort to improve your appearance, you find that your opinion of yourself becomes more positive," says mental health counselor Fred Silverstone, writing for older men in the Harvard Health Letter. Of course, his comment applies just as well to women.

3. *Pace yourself.* This essential insight comes from Toni Bernhard, who has created a plethora of helpful books and blogs on coping with chronic pain. Many of her insights apply also to aging. One of her helpful suggestions is the 50 percent rule: Decide what you can comfortably do, and then do just 50 percent of it. I would add: Prioritize what matters most, and just do that.

4. *Accept that both despair and joy will be part of the aging journey.* The losses of aging do take their toll. But surprisingly, research has documented that there is a steady rise in happiness among people over 50, despite problems of illness and aging. That's because, in the words of author and therapist Mary Pipher: "Many of us have learned that happiness is a skill and a choice. We don't need to look at our horoscopes to know how our day will go. We know how to create a good day."

5. *Approach the moment with a wholehearted attitude.* Cultivate the habit of opening up to the present moment and appreciating it. Even difficult moments can be savored. Mary Pipher again: "As we walk out of a friend's funeral, we can smell wood smoke in the air and taste snowflakes on our tongues."

6. *Reframe your* **problems** *as* **challenges**. This simple technique can immediately reduce stress and set your inner creative problem-solver into motion. For example, sample the difference between, "I have a problem with my husband," and "I have a challenge with my husband."

7. *Make time your friend.* I've learned that the passage of time—even five minutes—may change your pain level and even how you feel about your life in general. In this way, it resembles what we say about the weather in my hometown: "You don't like the weather? Just wait a minute." The ancient wisdom of "This, too, shall pass" still applies.

8. *Find a level of exercise that works for you.* A boatload of research tells us this: No amount of exercise, however small, is ever wasted. Whether in the form of standing up and stretching, household chores, or formal exercise, studies demonstrate numerous physical and mental health benefits of exercise, even in small bits. Since I'm an exercise cheerleader, it is ironic that I have not

been able to exercise in my usual way, and that is why I recommend that you:

9. *Find replacements for any activities you must curtail or stop.* While afflicted with heel pain, I've had to stop walking. But I've discovered that I can use a stationary bike or work out with weights while standing in place on a thick yoga mat.

10. *Connect with others, even in small ways.* It's not surprising that friends and family can be extremely helpful in lifting your spirits, but I've learned that acquaintances and even relative strangers can also be good companions on your journey. For example, I've gotten to know a variety of people at my physical therapy center. Chatting with them always gives me a lift and helps the time on that stationary bike go by more quickly. Because of my own experiences, I was interested to read recent research indicating that brief interactions with strangers can give you a mood boost. Even more evocative, this research "suggests that a happy life is made up of a high frequency of positive events, and even small positive experiences make a difference."

11. *Find a "purpose project."* Research strongly indicates the value of a sense of purpose for older adults. Benefits include better health and longevity, among others. Your purpose can be as personal as taking care of grandchildren or as complex as a social justice or a community project.

12. *Treat yourself to small pleasures.* Given that small positive experiences make for a happier life, as discussed above in #10, figure out how to include more of those experiences in your day. That's where treats come in. Treats do not necessarily have to be food treats. They can be exercise "snacks," cultural events, TV shows, books, fun conversations, and other small pleasures.

13. *Appreciate your age and the life that you've experienced.* When you think about it, it's really amazing to be on Planet Earth and to live a life here. Think of your age as an accomplishment, not as a liability.

14. *Find G.O.D.* Although I'm not religious, I find that having a spiritual orientation can be invaluable. In my case, I realized that I needed to focus on G.O.D. G.O.D. is my personal shorthand for "Gratitude Over Despair." Physical and psychological pain make it harder to be grateful. In the face of health troubles, I had to approach gratitude with deliberate intention, actively focusing on cultivating the "gratitude attitude."

In addition to this list, I'm sure you know to practice these common-sense actions: Eat right, get plenty of sleep, laugh a lot, and practice self-care. See a therapist if you feel depressed or call the Suicide Hotline (800-273-8255) if need be.

Refilling the Cart

In a way, I've been lucky that I've had to cope with a swarm of small problems rather than face one or more huge, devastating ones. My experience has been like a vaccination that may better prepare me when the bigger and stronger "viruses" come along. Hopefully my "coping immune system" has been activated.

Since I don't think anyone can live well with an empty cart, I see this list of 14 items as a way to lay in new supplies. I intend to pay particular attention to the idea of creating or noticing as many small positive experiences as I can in my day.

What items do you need for *your* cart?

© Meg Selig. Posted Sep 04, 2019, on psychologytoday.com.

References

Harvard Men's Health Watch, "Regain Your Confidence," June 2019, Harvard Health Publishing.

Pipher, M., "The Joy of Being a Woman in Her 70s." New York Times, 1/12/2019.

Neff, K. (2011). *Self-Compassion*. NY: HarperCollins.

Bernhard, T. Pacing: The Chronically Ill Person's Best Friend. Psychologytoday.com, June 15, 2016.

Nicolaus, P. "Want to Feel Happier Today? Try Talking to a Stranger." NPR, July 26, 2019.

One Small Spark:

✳

Maya Angelou's Complaint Department

"Sister, there are people who went to sleep all over the world last night, poor and rich and white and black, but they will never wake again. Sister, those who expected to rise did not, their beds became their cooling boards, and their blankets became their winding sheets. And those dead folks would give anything, anything at all for just five minutes of this weather or ten minutes of that plowing that person was grumbling about. So you watch yourself about complaining, Sister. What you're supposed to do when you don't like a thing is change it. If you can't change it, change the way you think about it. Don't complain."

—**Maya Angelou, Wouldn't Take Nothing for My Journey Now**

CHAPTER 29

NINE WAYS TO FIND YOUR PURPOSE AS YOU AGE

"Sooner or later I'm going to die, but I'm not going to retire."
—Margaret Mead

Surveys show that older people are happier people. But getting older is not a bed of roses. Eventually, the losses pile up. Friends, family members, or partners may die. You may acquire one or more chronic illnesses or become disabled. You may feel that your choices are narrowing.

Fortunately, there are still ways to find meaning in your life despite these losses. "Fortunately," because recent research reveals that living with a sense of purpose—acting in accord with your most cherished values and goals—has numerous benefits for both physical and mental health. For example, feeling that you have a purpose decreases your chance of premature death, according to a study of almost 7000 adults between the ages of 51 and 61. Amazingly, those without a sense of purpose were almost twice as likely to die in the four years of the study.

Other studies show that a sense of purpose promotes healthy behaviors and is associated with better physical and mental health outcomes. A 2019 study by a team of British researchers found that a sense of purpose also promoted happiness and a sense of well-being among adults 50- 90. The same researchers observed that older adults with a sense of purpose were more likely to have close friendships, enjoy the arts, practice healthy habits, and experience less chronic pain and illness. A recent study of seniors in a retirement community suggests that a sense of purpose might even alleviate loneliness.

According to an NPR report, it doesn't matter what your purpose is as long as you have one. But where do you look to find your unique purpose as you age?

Nine Paths to Purpose

For part of the answer, I returned to a favorite book: Viktor Frankl's, *Man's Search for Meaning*. In this short, powerful book, Frankl describes his daily experiences and observations while a prisoner in the concentration camps of Nazi Germany. There he developed his beliefs about what can sustain the desire to live even under the most inhumane and desperate circumstances.

Frankl observed that those inmates who had a sense of purpose were more likely to survive the degrading conditions of the camp. While the rigors of aging in no way compare to life in a concentration camp, they have in common the need to find meaningful goals when life gets rough.

Below are nine paths to purpose that can be helpful to anyone at any age, but they are especially relevant to older adults. I've drawn on Frankl's work for #1, #2, and #9. The ninth path may not strike you as particularly cheerful, but I think you'll find it bracing and even inspiring in its own way. By the way, you don't have to choose just one path. You might find yourself following each of the nine paths in turn, even in just one day.

1. Work mission.

Some older adults continue to work at a paid job that they love to do. Others use retirement as an opportunity to try out a second career. Still others just get any job, because earning an income is either necessary or a source of independence and pride. Many older adults find meaning in unpaid work such as volunteer work, personal projects, or home improvement.

One reason Frankl was motivated to survive the daily torment of the camps was because of a book he wanted to finish. Although he was forced to relinquish his manuscript when he entered the camp, he wrote his key ideas on scraps of paper and stuffed them in his pockets. After his liberation from the camps, he wrote that book and many others.

If you are no longer motivated by traditional work goals, however, you could find your particular purpose in one of the motivators below.

2. Love and friendship.

Finding meaning in the love of another person is an inspiring motivator. For example, Frankl was able to survive the camps in part by imagining a future reunion with his wife. Many older people find meaning in relationships with spouses, friends, children, and grandchildren and in taking care of beloved others.

3. Compassion for others.

Compassion and concern for others may protect against feelings of meaninglessness, according to a 2020 study. As one senior said, "If you're feeling lonely, then go out and do something for somebody else." Even making brief connections with relative strangers—acknowledging their presence, wishing them a good day, giving a compliment—can be a source both of meaning and happiness. Listening to someone with an open mind, reaching out to someone who may be lonely, or sending a card can provide good cheer to someone who is down in the dumps.

4. Small joys and pleasures.

But what if you don't have some lofty-sounding "purpose project" in your life? Just learning to appreciate small pleasures is a habit worth cultivating. Noticing a bird or plant outside your window, having a warming cup of coffee, exchanging hugs—these tiny moments when noticed and absorbed provide a source of satisfaction to both body and brain.

According to the "Bold School" newsletter of the *Washington Post,* researchers have studied people in Okinawa, Japan, where people live longer than anywhere in the world. Researchers attributed this longevity to the practice of "ikigai:" "This 'sense of a life worth living' includes looking for joy in small things, being present and creating a harmonious atmosphere."

5. Staying strong and healthy.

You won't be able to accomplish much if you lack energy and strength. And just staying strong to perform the normal activities of daily living is an accomplishment in itself, because it means that you can still be independent. Take walks, go to the gym, get a personal trainer, eat right—you know what to do!

6. Creative projects and play.

Creative activities, humor, and play of all sorts can provide a sense of purpose for many people. Hobbies, sports, and experiences such as art, travel, music, nature, reading, and culture can touch us deeply and enlarge our capacity for empathy. They may also reduce symptoms of chronic pain and worry by making life more enjoyable. Expressing your identity through art or actions is a way to be happy, a way to affirm who you are, and a way to find purpose.

7. Contributing to the repair and improvement of the world—or at least your corner of it.

Making a contribution to your society is a wonderful way to find a purpose greater than yourself. There are an infinite number of ways to do this. I have several friends who write letters-to-the-editor on a regular basis. Other people take up a social justice cause that is meaningful to them. Some people find a unique niche—for example, the skillful person whose mission is to help with the DIY projects of hapless neighbors and friends.

8. Leaving a legacy.

By a "legacy" I mean writing a will to ensure the smooth passage of your assets to your children or other heirs. But I also mean contributing to your family or to the world in many of the ways listed above. Answering the question, "What kind of gifts do I want to leave to the world before I die?" may even be an effective way to guide you toward your current purpose.

9. Bearing suffering with grace, courage, and dignity.

Counter-intuitive as it may sound, meeting the challenges of aging with acceptance and courage might become a mission in itself. Frankl's insight that enduring suffering could provide purpose in life was a mind-opener for me. He writes, for example, of life in the camps, that, "the hopelessness of our struggle did not detract from its dignity and its meaning." (Frankl emphasizes that suffering is not necessary to find meaning, only that meaning is possible in spite of suffering.)

How could you apply Frankl's insight to your life? You might decide to...

- Be a good role model for your children and others even when your life is painful.
- Focus on gratitude—what you do have rather than what you don't.

- Demonstrate courage by accepting what you cannot change.

I am not sure I will be able to do any of these things, but I think the awareness that I have a choice about how to deal with pain and suffering as I age will be helpful in itself. It is a revelation to realize that learning to cope with a tough situation creatively can become a source of meaning in itself.

Final Thoughts

The experiences of aging—in fact, of life in general—can be bitter, sweet, tender, or tough. How will you react to them? You might find it useful to remember these words of Frankl's: "...in the final analysis, it becomes clear that the sort of person the prisoner became was the result of an inner decision, and not the result of camp influences alone." What kind of person do you want to be as you age? Can you make an "inner decision" that will guide you?

© Meg Selig, 2020. Posted Feb 02, 2020, psychologytoday.com.

References

Gordon, M. "What's Your Purpose? Finding a Sense of Meaning in Life is Linked to Health." NPR, 2019.

Frankl, V.E. (2006). Man's Search for Meaning. Boston: Beacon Press, p. 105. (First published in English in 1959), pp. 66, 83, 105, 111, 113.

"Lonely in a Crowd: Overcoming Loneliness with Acceptance and Wisdom." ScienceDaily, 1.10.2020.

OTHER VOICES:
Aging and Purpose

"It's never too late—in fiction or in life—to revise."

—Nancy Thayer

"There must be a goal at every stage of life! There must be a goal!"

—Maggie Kuhn, founder of the Gray Panthers

"The real problem is that there's a tendency to associate ageing with loss and decline and things that aren't desirable. But experiencing all that there is to experience in life—whether that's at the age of ten or thirty or fifty or eighty—is what life is all about."

—S. Jay Olshansky, Gerontologist

"For the unlearned, old age is winter; for the learned, it is the season of the harvest."

—Hasidic Saying

"The longer I live the more beautiful life becomes."

—Frank Lloyd Wright

PART V

DEATH AND OTHER ENDINGS

CHAPTER 30

NINE WAYS TO EASE THE FEAR OF DEATH

What are the most helpful ways to cope with the reality of one's own death?

Accepting the Reality of Death

How did you react when you first discovered you would someday die?

I can well remember my outrage—yes, *outrage*—when I learned at the age of 5 or so that my life was not going to last forever. Here I was, just realizing who I was and rejoicing in my newly-discovered self, only to find out that I was already on the road to oblivion.

My father comforted me with the words that many parents no doubt use: "You won't have to worry about that for a long, long time."

Although I can remember feeling slightly mollified by his comment, there was a part of my younger self that could not be comforted. Death would indeed come for me someday. Still,

I got my father's message. Yes, maybe I could put death off for a long, long time.

I'm now in middle old age and continuing to use the defense of denial. "I could have 20 more good years," I tell myself. "I won't have to worry for a long, long time." Still, at my age, I think I need a bigger boat of strategies.

What are the most helpful ways to cope with the reality of death? Those who believe in an afterlife have a built-in buffer against the fear of death. But for the rest of us, are there any ways that psychology can help lessen the dread of our own death?* The following nine methods may be helpful.

1. Use the fear of death as motivation to lengthen your life by practicing healthy habits.

Exercise. Healthy eating. Enough sleep. Good relationships. Being in nature. Taking breaks. Flossing. All these healthy habits contribute to a longer, healthier life and to a happier one, too, according to an ever-increasing body of research.

In addition, healthy habits increase the odds that you will avoid the worst ravages of aging and even keep some spring in your step until the end. Make your "healthspan" as long as your lifespan.

2. Get older and become less fearful.

When I was in my mid-50s, I had another talk with my parents about death. My father said, "Now that we are older, we are less afraid of dying." And my mother nodded in agreement. I regret that I cannot remember the rest of our conversation. *Why* was he less afraid? *Why* did they bring it up? I'll never know, thanks to my anxiety about discussing the subject.

But now that I am older, I do fear death less myself. Psychologists tell us that prolonged exposure to something— even to the idea of death—helps us adapt to it. A friend's mother put it this way: "If you have an elephant in your living room, you eventually get used to it."

The battle against the aches and pains of daily living also takes its toll. As author Mary Roach says, "I don't fear death so much as I fear its prologues: loneliness, decrepitude, pain, debilitation, depression, senility. After a few years of those, I imagine death presents like a holiday at the beach."

To ease the fear of death, just get older.

3. Open up to gratitude.

I would like to believe that my father and mother had also enjoyed such a good life that they were ready to let it go, like guests who have feasted at the Thanksgiving table, realize they are satisfied, and need no more. Maybe they felt like Leonardo da Vinci, who said: "As a well-spent day brings happy sleep, so a life well spent brings happy death."

Focusing on the positive events and people in your life can help you replace fearfulness with gratitude. The gratitude attitude, moreover, brings countless benefits to those who cultivate it. Research tells us that gratitude is closely related to happiness, a sense of purpose, and reduced stress. The famous "Three Good Things" exercise and related activities have an amazing effect on happiness, even when practiced for a short period of time.

4. Create a legacy.

By "legacy," I mean several things. First, there is the priceless legacy of preparing a will and other related documents. Yes, it's tedious. But by specifying exactly who should get what, you can do your part to avoid wounding fights within the family that leave undying hard feelings (pun intended).

By "legacy," I also mean the actions, words, and deeds that you leave behind after you die. The memories others have of you are a type of life extension. That means that if you need to apologize to certain people or to express your love and gratitude to certain others, now is the time to do it.

Finally, you might consider giving the gift of death cleaning as part of your legacy. Yes, I did say "death cleaning," a Swedish custom that I have adopted. (More in the next chapter.) Death cleaning involves cleaning up after yourself before you leave this Earth—organizing, sorting, tossing, or giving away your possessions and keepsakes. Without consciously engaging in "death cleaning," I've noticed that many older people are preoccupied with cleaning their basements or attics. I think they are instinctively doing one last favor for their children by making life—and death—a little easier for them.

Once you have prepared your legacy, the sound of the footsteps of death may evoke less terror. You are ready.

5. Keep your purpose top of mind.

Psychologist Sonja Lyubomirsky, writing in *The Myths of Happiness*, cites research supporting the idea that living with a sense of purpose is the best way to cope with the fear of death. As she points out, finding purpose involves actions that link you to something greater than yourself—alleviating the suffering of others, imparting your values to the next generation, creating work of lasting value, or investing in the community, to give just a few examples.

Lyubomirsky suggests this simple process for doing what matters most: "...Take at least one step each week in the direction that helps you attain purpose in your life and secures your legacy." (For help in defining your purpose(s), see "Nine Ways to Find Your Purpose as You Age.")

6. Express your creativity.

Expressing who you are through creative activities is one of the best ways to feel alive, as well as to create a legacy for others. And by "creativity," I do not mean just artistic expression. Everyone has a creative side, whether they express it through woodworking, leadership, public speaking, establishing a business or charity, educating children, or almost any human endeavor. Anything you have made—including pottery, photo albums, letters, books, videos, blogs, fabric arts, paintings, or records of other professional accomplishments—can become precious mementos for your children and grandchildren.

7. Let the knowledge of death help you appreciate the sweetness of life.

> "It is from some obscure recognition of the fact of death that life draws its final sweetness."
> —Alexander Smith

Scottish essayist Alexander Smith wrote in 1863 that, "It is from some obscure recognition of the fact of death that life draws its final sweetness."

In fact, since turning 65, I have experienced strange moments of transcendent happiness. Perhaps Mother Nature provides these moments to all creatures in autumn, as we go about gathering nectar in the final stages of life.

Whether or not that is true, we can choose to be mindful of the small things in life that bring pleasure and happiness. A good cup of coffee, a beautiful view, a robin in the yard—anyone can decide to become a master at noting and appreciating the tiny joys of life. This skill may even help you live longer. The Japanese elders of Okinawa who practice the art of *ikigai*, noticing small pleasures, are the longest-lived people on Earth. This mindful noticing will also bring you into the present moment, freeing you from past regrets or future worries.

8. Find social support and talk about your anxieties.

Reading between the lines of this blog, you can discern that discussing the subject of death with my parents, however awkward, nonetheless gave me permission to think about it, write about it, and begin to accept it. Talking to family members, therapists, or friends could serve the same purpose. "Death Cafes" have sprung up all over the world with the goal of presenting programs that help people talk about and prepare for death.

In general, social support—knowing that others care about you and have your back—can insulate you from all manner of ills as well as promote longevity, health, and happiness, according to research cited by Lyubomirsky. She describes emotionally supportive relationships as "the single best way to prepare for a future fateful diagnosis or any kind of tragedy or crisis."

9. Indulge in a little death humor.

Death wins in the end, but at least we can poke fun at it along the way. Even cornball jokes can help. That reminds me—do you know why life is like a roll of toilet paper? Because the closer you get to the end, the faster it goes.

Final Thoughts

When it's time for me to go, I hope I am able to use these techniques to ease my end-of-life fear or at least make the fact of death a little more bearable. I hope this blog has given you some comforting and useful ideas, too. Perhaps at some point, you might agree with the Harry Potter character who said, "After all, to the well-organized mind, death is but the next great adventure." I'm not sure I could adopt that point of view, but I can relate to this wise saying from the Buddha: "Even death is not to be feared by one who has lived wisely."

In other words, to lessen your fear of death, live a good life.

© *Meg Selig, 2020.*

*Note that I am limiting this blog to facing one's own death in the fullness of time. Early deaths, deaths of beloved others, and especially deaths of children and young people present special challenges and hardships. Also, if you are experiencing suicidal thoughts and/or depression, contact a mental health professional or call the National Suicide Prevention Hotline number for resources, 800-273-8255.

References

Lyubomirsky, S. (2013) *The Myths of Happiness.* (NY: Penguin Books), p. 205 ff.

Perry, S. "You're Going to Die: Three Ways to Lessen Your Dread," April 14, 2019: psychologytoday.com.

Solomon, S., Greenberg, J., and Pyszczynski, T. (2015). *The Worm at the Core: On the Role of Death in Life.* NY: Random House. p. 210 ff.

CHAPTER 31

CAN'T GET YOURSELF TO DECLUTTER? TRY "DEATH CLEANING"

"Death cleaning is not sad."
— Margareta Magnusson,
The Gentle Art of Swedish
Death Cleaning

An Unusual Motivator for Cleaning Up As You Age

Have you resolved to declutter part of your home or office in the next few weeks? If so, what is your motivator? Maybe you...

- Value order and want to be able to find the things you need more easily.
- Value beauty and want your surroundings to be pleasing to the eye.
- Value simplicity. You like to "have only what you need and nothing that you don't," to paraphrase a country song.
- Value clear thinking. You have realized that an orderly environment can help you think and work better.

- Value the inner calm that you feel when your surroundings are tidy and clean.

All of these are worthwhile motivators.

But here's a motivator for cleaning up, sorting, and organizing that I bet you haven't fully considered: **Death**.

In *The Gentle Art of Swedish Death Cleaning*, a short book by Swedish artist Margareta Magnusson, you are encouraged to practice "death cleaning." (There is an actual word for "death cleaning" in Swedish: *"dostadning."*) The goal of death cleaning is both to get your things in order before you die and to live better right now. The subtitle, "How to Free Yourself and Your Family from a Lifetime of Clutter," expresses the perspective of the book. While the phrase "death cleaning" may sound macabre at first, in Magnusson's hands, the job of death cleaning can become a matter-of-fact and even a light-hearted endeavor. "Death cleaning is not sad," Magnusson proclaims in chapter 1.

"Death Cleaning" Defined

"Death cleaning" can refer to cleaning up after the death of another person or to cleaning up your own things prior to your own death. When you decide to do a bit of death cleaning for yourself, you might sort your possessions, donating some to charity, tossing others, gifting a few things to various important people, and keeping other things for yourself. Death cleaning does not have to be a chore; you can go at your own pace, delighting in your possessions and the memories they evoke. As you sort and re-organize, you learn to manage your everyday life with greater ease, creating time to do more of what you want.

Magnusson, who describes her age as "somewhere between eighty and one hundred years old," describes two additional reasons for death cleaning. One is to spare your loved ones the task of cleaning up your junk after you've died. When you must death-clean as a result of someone else's death, it can be a burdensome chore. It is an act of unselfish kindness to "clean up after yourself" before you leave the earth. Second, you want to spare yourself the embarrassment of having your loved ones come upon journals, photos, letters, and objects that you would rather not have them see.

Although I'd never heard the term "death cleaning" until I read this book, I must confess I've had occasion to think about those two motivators. Recently I was cleaning up after re-modeling my study and came upon a journal I'd written in my 20's. Within those pages I revealed…well…all sorts of cringe-worthy things that I would never want anyone in my own family—or in anyone else's family, for that matter—to know about.

I shredded that journal. Believe me, nothing of historical worth was destroyed, and my privacy was protected.

Suggestions

Magnusson favors a gradual process of cleaning up, taking time to assess whether an object would make you or anyone else happier. Among her many observations, I particularly liked these:

"Mess is an unnecessary source of irritation."
"If you find yourself repeatedly having the same problem, fix it!"
"If you don't like something, get rid of it."

She advises that we all learn to enjoy things without owning them.

When to Death Clean

As a woman between the ages of sixty and eighty, I realize it is time to think about death cleaning. Magnusson recommends starting at about age 65. Personally, I think any time is a good time, especially if you need to whisk away any secret, dangerous, or embarrassing objects (see above). And it can be helpful to remind yourself now and then that you are mortal, so that you don't put things off that could make your life better or more meaningful in some way.

Finishing Touches

There are other "death cleaning" actions not mentioned in the book that are also vitally important. Make a will. Communicate your last wishes to your loved ones. Yes, those goals are difficult to carry out, but not doing so can also have enormous costs. And if you have pack-rat tendencies, consider hiring an organizing professional or seeing a therapist who specializes in hoarding.

Magnusson's little book may help you find the motivator for decluttering that has so far eluded you. And one unanticipated benefit of her book is that it might make you feel just a shade more comfortable with the idea of your eventual demise.

© Meg Selig. Posted Feb 06, 2018, on psychologytoday.com

Reference

Magnusson, Margareta, "The Gentle Art of Swedish Death Cleaning: How to Free Yourself and Your Family from a Lifetime of Clutter," (New York: Scribner), 2018.

CHAPTER 32

THREE GOOD THINGS ABOUT DEATH: AN EXPERIMENT

Could a gratitude exercise help someone face death? I try it out.

As I've gotten older, I think about my own death more often. It's a shocking thought. I never fully realized that when the ancient philosopher said, "All men are mortal," he was referring to ME. Now I know that he was.

Of course, I could live for another 30 years or step off the curb the wrong way and die within the hour. But I will die sometime. I am trying to make peace with this idea, but I can't quite wrap my mind around it. Here today, gone tomorrow? The thought makes me shudder.

I am just enjoying life too much to think of The End. Like many older people, I've learned to cherish and savor each day. I don't even care if the weather is bad or good. It's all good to me. Because, as the old song says, "I'm still here." And I don't want to go, thank you very much.

One day it occurred to me that perhaps I could use the "Three Good Things" exercise to help myself deal with the "Big D." This exercise is a well-researched way to increase personal happiness and gratitude. In just one of many experiments, researchers asked college students to write down three good things that had happened to them each day for one week, along with their interpretations of *why* those things had happened. The results were amazing. The experimental group saw their happiness levels soar, not just immediately but for the next six months. This was after only one week of practicing gratitude!

Similar gratitude exercises have yielded similar benefits. Recently I learned that Yale University's most popular course ever is Psych 157, "Psychology and the Good Life." And what do these students do for happiness homework? "The three good things" exercise. (Actually, they have to write down five good things they are grateful for—but this is Yale. They are over-achievers.)

I started doing this exercise myself back in 2009, when I discovered the research. I was so impressed that I included it in my book *Changepower! 37 Secrets to Habit Change Success,* because it turns out that happiness and gratitude can help you maintain a desired habit change. I've continued to count my blessings ever since. For me, the benefits are legion—the gratitude attitude, more happiness, a healthier perspective on my problems, and even an increased sense of personal competence.

But would this exercise help me feel better about death?

When I say "death," by the way, I am not referring to "dying," a process that is surely fraught with poignancy at best and pain and suffering at worst. I am also putting to one side all religious views of what may or may not happen in the afterlife, and just assuming that I will become, well, dust. I'm also not referring to the loss of a beloved person or to anyone else's death, especially the deaths of children or of those cut off in their prime by war, disease, or pestilence. These are tragic events, plain and simple.

By "death," I mean the state of not being alive any more. For me, would there be anything good about being dead? Could I possibly come up with at least three good things about that?

Of course I can. Here they are:

The first good thing about death is that I will never have to be on hold for or speak to anyone at a call center ever again. If there are call centers in the afterlife, then I will know for sure that I'm in Hell. Recently, however, I discovered something worse than a call center: Having to go online and solve your problem all by yourself. Maybe Hell is self-service.

The second good thing about death is that there will no longer be a need for body maintenance. By "body maintenance," I mean doctors and dentists appointments and all the things you must do to your face, skin, and teeth every morning and night just to stay healthy. In death, you can let everything go. And it will. (Of course, I could also argue that I'm lucky to have doctors and dentists to take care of me. You see how the gratitude attitude seeps into your bones?)

The third and best good thing: I would finally sleep through the night. In the last 15 years, I don't think I've had one night of uninterrupted sleep. As you age, your bladder gradually shrinks to the size of a sunflower seed. I'm so grateful when I only awaken once and can get back to sleep in a reasonable amount of time. More often, I'm up two or three times a night. In death, my sleep would most definitely not be interrupted. True, it will be a long, long night. I guess that's why they call it "eternal rest."

And the other good things...so many possibilities! When I'm gone, I certainly won't miss the devastating crises of life or even its minor inconveniences, such as home repairs, computer breakdowns, and car troubles, not to mention the endless struggle of adapting to new technologies. But these are minor hassles. All in all, I love life, and, assuming I could be relatively healthy, well-off, in contact with friends and family, and free of most of the ravages of old age, I could figure out ways to be happy.

While I am wishing, I'd like to make it clear that I desire both immortality AND eternal youth. I don't want to make the mistake of the woman in Greek mythology who asked the gods for eternal life for her lover but forgot to specify that he remain young as well. He ended up much like a cicada. Of course, that's where we're all going anyway.

Bottom line: Although I feel a little better about the Great Beyond, I can't claim to accept the idea of my own death just yet, even after considering some of its benefits. But what I *can* do is feel grateful for my lucky life and for every single moment I have left in this crazy, amazing world.

OTHER VOICES:
On Death and Dying

"You only live once, but if you do it right, once is enough."

—Mae West

*"I know that I shall not live very long. But I wonder, is that sad?
Is a celebration more beautiful because it lasts longer?
And my life is a celebration, a short, intense celebration."*

—Paula Modersohn-Becker, painter

*"There is no good reason why we should not develop and
change until the last day we live."*

—Karen Horney

*"Humans will die like all living things do, but we have
the added burden of knowing that we will."*

—S. Jay Olshansky

*"In the depths of winter, I finally learned that within me
there lay an invincible summer."*

—Albert Camus

"There is always something left to love."

—Lorraine Hansbury, *A Raisin in the Sun*

SELECT BIBLIOGRAPHY

Applewhite, A. (2016). *This Chair Rocks: A Manifesto Against Ageism.* NY: Celadon Books.

Aronson, L. (2019) *Elderhood: Redefining Aging, Transforming Medicine, Reimagining Life.* NY: Bloomsbury Publishing.

Bernhard, T. (2020) *How to Be Sick: Your Pocket Companion.* Somerville, MA: Wisdom Publications.

Carstensen, L. (2011). *A Long Bright Future: Happiness, Health, and Financial Security in an Age of Increased Longevity.* NY: Broadway Books.

Casner, Steve (2017). *Careful: A User's Guide to Our Injury-Prone Minds.* NY: Riverhead Books

Chodron, Pema (2013). *How to Meditate.* Boulder: Sounds True.

Clear, J. (2018). *Atomic Habits: Tiny Changes, Remarkable Results.* NY: Avery

Cohen, G. (2005). *The Positive Power of the Aging Brain.* NY: Basic Books.

Douglas, S. (2020). *In Our Prime: How Older Women Are Reinventing the Road Ahead.* New York: WW Norton.

Emmons, R.A. (2007). *Thanks! How Practicing Gratitude Can Make You Happier.* Boston: Houghton Mifflin.

Frankl, V. (2006). *Man's Search for Meaning.* Boston: Beacon Press.

Fogg, BJ (2020). *Tiny Habits: The Small Changes That Change Everything.* Boston: Houghton Mifflin Harcourt.

Greenberg, M. (2016). *The Stress-Proof Brain.* Oakland, CA: New Harbinger.

Kay, K. & Shipman, C. (2014). The *Confidence Code.* NY: HarperCollins.

Lyubamirsky, S. (2014). *The Myths of Happiness.* NY: Penguin Books.

Magnusson, M. (2018). *The Gentle Art of Swedish Death-Cleaning: How to Free Yourself and Your Family from a Lifetime of Clutter. NY: Scribner*

Ornish M.D., D. (2019) *Undo It!: How Simple Lifestyle Changes Can Reverse Most Chronic Diseases.* NY: Ballantine.

Pipher, M. (2019). *Women Rowing North: Navigating Life's Currents and Flourishing As We Age.* NY: Bloomsbury Publishing.

Rauch, Jonathan (2018). *The Happiness Curve: Why Life Gets Better After 50.* NY: Picador.

Schlossberg, N. (2010). *Revitalizing Retirement: Reshaping Your Identity, Relationships, and Purpose.* APA: Washington, D.C.

Unruh, A.C. (2015). *Coffee is Cheaper than Therapy.* St. Louis: Forest Green.

Wykle, M.L. et al, eds. (2005). *Successful Aging Through the Life Span.* NY: Springer Publishing Company.

THE GRATITUDE LIST

"Give credit where credit is due" has always been one of my favorite mottoes. Credit for this book is due to numerous people:

- My writing partner and friend, the amazing Helen Gennari.
- My daughter Elizabeth Selig for her wisdom, kindness and humor. And to my son-in-law Trond Kristiansen and my granddaughter Eloise. Eloise, just thinking about you makes me smile!
- My union, the National Education Association, which has fought for the rights of educators, enabling me to retire at 62 and embark on a new career as a writer. Reader, may you, too, have a "defined-benefit" pension someday! More I cannot wish you.
- My friend and colleague in self-publishing, Rebecca (Becky) Garrison.
- My various friends and supporters, especially my long-time friends Jane Klopfenstein, Patsy O'Connell, Elizabeth Powell, and Susan Waugh. Colleagues Howard Rosenthal and Ank Ankenbrand were essential to my professional

progress. Thank you for your support.

- My partner Brian Carr and his daughter Rachel Carr. Thanks to both for the wonderful dinners!
- My "blog friends" who have stayed on my "blog notification list" for 10 years and counting, including many valued friends from high school.
- My sister Kate Kimelman, editor, problem-solver, brainstormer, and sympathetic ear.
- To the memory of my parents. I appreciate you now more than ever and think about you daily.
- The editors at psychologytoday.com, along with Sussex Publishers, LLC, and my fellow and sister bloggers who are kind enough to share their wisdom in the "Green Room."
- The good people at JetLaunch who put up with my endless questions and requests. Thank you for your patience and good work!
- Dana Bliss, my editor at Routledge/Taylor & Francis, who brought my first book, *Changepower! 37 Secrets to Habit Change Success,* to life. Thank you for your faith in me, Dana.
- Anyone who writes personal essays owes a debt of gratitude to Nora Ephron, whether they know it or not. I know it. Thank you, Nora Ephron, and rest in peace.

I am so grateful for all of you! Thank you!

—Meg Rashbaum Selig

ABOUT THE AUTHOR

Meg Selig was 65 when her first book, *Changepower! 37 Secrets to Habit Change Success,* was published by Routledge in 2009. In 2010, she was invited to blog for *Psychology Today* at psychologytoday.com where she continues to write the "Changepower" blog. She focuses on the "three H's," health, happiness, and habits, along with healthy aging, mindful living, motivation, and confidence.

Selig earned her M.A. Ed. in Counseling at Washington University in St. Louis in 1974. Prior to retiring from fulltime work at age 62, Selig was a licensed professional counselor (LPC) and national certified counselor (NCC) in various school settings. She began her career as a counselor in elementary, middle, and high schools, then "graduated" to the college setting. She worked at St. Louis Community College for over 20 years, continuing to work part-time after she retired.

As a latecomer to the world of writing, Selig has a special understanding of the challenges facing older workers and those in retirement as they seek to find meaning and purpose in their later years. She is encouraged by the fact that while she was a "late bloomer" as an author, she did, in fact, bloom. Her hope is that others will find new ways to express themselves and contribute to others in their Golden Years as well.

Now in her mid-70's, Selig is grateful for her experiences as a daughter, mother, grandmother, wife, divorcee, worker, partner, and friend. These experiences have all contributed to her perspectives on youth and aging.

Selig lives in St. Louis, Missouri, and enjoys life with her long-time partner, Brian Carr.

● ● ●

The author's popular blog, "Changepower," is hosted by *Psychology Today*: www.psychologytoday.com/us/blog/changepower.

The author website is: www.megselig.com.

For permissions or questions, email the author at: megselig@hotmail.com

The author's Facebook author page is: www.facebook.com/megselig

You can follow her on Twitter at this handle: @MegSelig1

One Small Spark:

One Small Favor: Pass It On!

Did you enjoy and benefit from this book? If so, please buy a copy for a friend. Your generous act could "spark" another person to create "silver years" that are more joyous, meaningful, and healthy.

Thank you for reading *Silver Sparks!*

NOTES

Made in the USA
Las Vegas, NV
27 December 2020